THE
QUICK
AND
THE
DEAD

Royalties from the sale of this book are pledged to the Palmerston North Rescue Helicopter. We live in a relatively far-flung and sparsely peopled country where access in an emergency can be difficult. The familiar beat of the helicopters of this magnificent service never fails to make us look up and wonder what has happened and upon what errand of mercy they are embarking. And when we do so it is with gratitude and also pride, too, for they are our people and it is our service. It is therefore fitting that these, our community stories of the quick and the dead, are devoted as a tribute to their ceaseless vigil.

CYNRIC TEMPLE-CAMP

THE QUICK AND THE DEAD

True stories of life and death
from a New Zealand pathologist

HarperCollins*Publishers*

HarperCollinsPublishers

First published in 2020
by HarperCollinsPublishers (New Zealand) Limited
Unit D1, 63 Apollo Drive, Rosedale, Auckland 0632, New Zealand
harpercollins.co.nz

Copyright © Cynric Temple-Camp 2020

Cynric Temple-Camp asserts the moral right to be identified as the author of this work. This work is copyright. All rights reserved. No part of this publication may be reproduced, copied, scanned, stored in a retrieval system, recorded, or transmitted, in any form or by any means, without the prior written permission of the publisher.

HarperCollinsPublishers
Unit D1, 63 Apollo Drive, Rosedale, Auckland 0632, New Zealand
Level 13, 201 Elizabeth Street, Sydney, NSW 2000, Australia
A 53, Sector 57, Noida, UP, India
1 London Bridge Street, London, SE1 9GF, United Kingdom
Bay Adelaide Centre, East Tower, 22 Adelaide Street West, 41st floor, Toronto,
   Ontario M5H 4E3, Canada
195 Broadway, New York NY 10007, USA

A catalogue record for this book is available from the National Library of New Zealand.

ISBN 978 1 7755 4151 6 (pbk)
ISBN 978 1 7754 9182 8 (ebook)

Cover design by Mark Campbell, HarperCollins Design Studio
Front cover image by shutterstock.com
Back cover image by Santi Nunez/Stocksy.com/2493706
Typeset in Bembo Std by Kirby Jones
Printed and bound in Australia by McPherson's Printing Group
The papers used by HarperCollins in the manufacture of this book are a natural, recyclable product made from wood grown in sustainable plantation forests. The fibre source and manufacturing processes meet recognised international environmental standards, and carry certification.

In memory of Jason Chase.
The dead teach the living.

CONTENTS

Prologue	The Quick—	1
Chapter 1	My Bowels Will Be the Death of Me	9
Chapter 2	Troubles with the Liver	28
Chapter 3	The Creatures Within Us	49
Chapter 4	Earth to Earth, Ashes to Ashes, Dust to Dust	70
Chapter 5	The Meat-Eaters	88
Chapter 6	Line of Duty	113
Chapter 7	The Cancer Wakes	132
Chapter 8	Death at the Chicken Ranch	157
Chapter 9	Shotguns in the Manawatu	180
Chapter 10	Unfortunate Deaths	204
Chapter 11	We've Made a Dreadful Mistake	221
Chapter 12	Perils in the Bush	246
Chapter 13	In My Considered Opinion	273
Chapter 14	Fit to Burst	295
Epilogue	—and the Dead	320

PROLOGUE

The Quick—

'Hold off the earth a while
Till I have caught her once more in mine arms.'
Laertes as he leaps into Ophelia's grave to embrace her body.
'Now pile your dust upon the Quick and the Dead.'
— William Shakespeare, *Hamlet* 5.1 233–235

'So I hear you're a pathologist?'

People often look at me uneasily as they say this. Perhaps they sense that, through me, the Horsemen of the Apocalypse are already circling them. They're right, but those deathly horses have nothing to do with me. They're always there, continually circling us all. I am only there to help pick up the pieces after they have visited.

People imagine the job of a pathologist is only to crudely carve up the dead, but it's not true. We spend most of our lives investigating, diagnosing and helping the 'quick', as the Bible calls people yet alive. Doctors are no different from anyone else:

we have different personalities. Some prefer personal contact with their patients and administering care to the living: they are, rightly, the front-room boys and girls of medicine.

That's not me.

From early on in my career, I decided I prefer the kind of 'hard' science that pathologists are involved with — observation, testing, the gathering of evidence, making deductions. Pathologists are the back-room boys and girls, searching for the scientific answers to the questions posed by disease and death.

When I was not even a year out from finishing my stint as a house surgeon and the ink on my diploma was barely dry, I landed a job as a general practitioner looking after the families of Rhodesian Air Force personnel. I was 24 years old and shaving once a day more from hope than need.

On my first day, I presented myself to Richard, the principal medical officer at New Sarum Air Force Station. He consulted his notes, and looked up at me speculatively from where he was sitting formally behind his desk. 'You can take over Mrs Bezuidenhout,' he said. 'It'll be good for you. Besides, we've all had our turn with her. Bloody woman!'

I narrowed my eyes.

'Why, Richard? What's wrong with Mrs Bezuidenhout?'

'It's "Sir" to you, not Richard. Or "Squadron Leader". I don't mind which.'

He looked more amused than annoyed that I had given him the opportunity to pull rank on me, and for good reason. He had only been a year or two ahead of me at medical school and wasn't even a specialist.

'She's completely loco,' he said. 'She's convinced her baby just stops breathing. She's always barging into the base hospital and disrupting our day's work schedule. She does it several times a week, in fact. And four times now in the middle of the night, I've rushed around to carry out an emergency resuscitation only to find a healthy boy sleeping peacefully. She's also got the civilian ambulance crews out a couple of times and now they've complained to the Base Commander. He's ordered me to sort her out, the bloody fool. Don't know what he thinks I can do about it.'

A broad smile crossed his face.

'So I'm telling you that you can do it.' He pointed at my chest. 'That's how the military works.'

It was supposed to be a hospital pass — no pun intended — but my interest was piqued. I was curious to meet the infant James Bezuidenhout and see whether I could spot something that my colleagues had missed. I didn't have to wait long for the opportunity, or much longer after that for another, and another.

Within a week, I too had had enough of panicked calls late at night. Each time, I examined the boy and found him normal in every way. I eventually had him tightly wrapped in a towel and pinned down by a nurse while I drew blood from his jugular vein, his mother looking on with her big, round eyes filled with horror and accusation.

She maintained the same intense stare as I explained to her that James's blood tests were all reassuringly normal. She made me feel distinctly uneasy. I wondered whether perhaps I should send her to a psychiatrist. I just didn't know what to do.

So it went for several months. James kept breathing as he always had and, far from dying, he met all his milestones, growing as any normal child should. It was a relief when I was deployed to the Forward Airfield at Kariba in the

Zambezi Valley for a couple of weeks. Even the bush war seemed preferable to meeting Mrs Bezuidenhout's baleful glare, day after day.

I hardly gave her a passing thought until my tour in the bush was over. But her name soon came up when I was doing a debrief with the elderly GP who had been called up to locum for me while I was away.

'It's all over with Mrs Bezuidenhout,' he said. 'It's all sorted out.'

'Oh!' I said. 'Has she emigrated?'

I had secretly been longing for this to happen. It was the only solution I could imagine.

'No. She came in to see me with young James. I took one look as she came through the door and said: "Young lady, you have got severe thyrotoxicosis. You need treatment right now."'

'Thyrotoxicosis?' I replied faintly.

'Yes,' he said, grinning. 'Graves' disease. You'll remember that from your textbooks, won't you? And you will have noticed her bulging eyes. She has typical thyroid exophthalmos.'

Thyroid exophthalmos. Bulging eyes! It all fitted. And all this time I thought she was just staring angrily at me.

'I started her on treatment and she's fine now,' he continued. 'She's sleeping well and no more high anxiety, thank God. That's all this whole saga was ever about. There never was anything wrong with her young lad, of course. Thyrotoxicosis makes you highly anxious, as you know, and James had just become the entire focus of her disease anxiety.'

'I missed it completely.' I sat there and stared at him. I felt a complete and useless idiot.

The grandfatherly old-timer slapped me on the back.

'Never mind, young fella. You'll learn the tricks soon enough. Always look at the whole story — the whole family and not just the single symptom the patient is complaining of — and one day, you'll become a fine GP.'

Maybe he was right, maybe he wasn't. I decided then and there that general practice wasn't for me. I think I always knew it, anyway, even as a medical student: I just didn't have the right stuff for that sort of job. Now I'm older, I still feel terrible I got it so wrong. I found Sheila Bezuidenhout to be a lovely lady once her runaway thyroid gland was tamed and I got to know her better. Inexplicably, she still stuck loyally to me as her GP of choice, despite my shameful failure to spot her diagnosis. That's more than I would have done.

No, I decided, I wasn't going to be a GP. I was going to get into a laboratory and become a pathologist. There would be no more Mrs Bezuidenhouts to bother me there.

I would do it just as soon as I could.

* * *

I did eventually become a pathologist, with a laboratory and a mortuary.

Wandering the laboratory one day soon after I had begun, I bumped into Colin Wilson, one of our surgeons. He was clearly on a mission.

'Could you put through Chandra Naik's colectomy as soon as possible?' he asked.

'Certainly. What's her story?'

'It's not really that urgent a specimen,' Colin explained, 'but it's bad news for her and the family, I'm afraid. She presented with typical bowel obstruction. Colicky pain, faeculent vomiting and dilated loops of small bowel filled with fluid and gas on plain X-ray. She had the works. I opened her up and it's a typical colon cancer, I'm sorry to say. It's right in the middle of the transverse colon. There is a large, hard cancer encircling the bowel and completely blocking the passage. Unfortunately it's already spread far and there are nodules of metastatic cancer dotted all around the mesentery of the colon. Nothing really that I could do to help her.'

Colin is a highly experienced and skilled general surgeon. Chandra was the mother of a respected colleague. She was visiting her son from India. This was absolutely the worst possible outcome. There was nothing man or medicine could do to save Chandra now. It would be a matter of palliative care for a few weeks or months, and then Chandra would surely die.

'I just did a limited local resection to relieve the blockage and make her comfortable until the end,' Colin said to me. 'With the obvious spread of the cancer, I thought there was no point in doing a more aggressive operation aimed at a cure.'

We duly dissected the resected length of colon in the lab and the tumour was exactly as Colin had described. It was a typical bowel cancer which had escaped and spread far and wide. I could see signs of necrosis as far away as her distant lymph nodes, the sure sign of an aggressive, malignant cancer.

The following day, I glanced down my microscope at a slide bearing a stained sample of the cancerous tissue.

I looked again. I couldn't believe what I was seeing.

I picked up the phone and called Colin.

'Colin,' I said. 'Chandra hasn't got cancer at all! She's got tuberculosis!'

There was a long, sceptical silence.

'Tuberculosis? But how? It looks exactly like a typical cicatricial bowel carcinoma! I've never heard of tuberculosis presenting this way.'

'It's a tuberculoma, a tumour but made up of tuberculous granulomas and scar tissue. It's not common, but TB can do this in any organ and present in virtually every possible way. The old physicians used to say that syphilis was the great mimic, but that's true of tuberculosis, too. And this is tuberculosis! There's no cancer!'

There was another pause, this one reflective.

'You know, a strange thing happened when I went out to explain to the family what I had found during the operation and my fears for her future. They took it well. In fact, they were quite serene. The Naiks are a strongly Christian family. It was almost as if they'd had a word from God. "She will be fine," they told me. "She will be cured." This was cancer, pure and simple, for my money. There was no hope at all. But now it turns out they were absolutely right. You have to admire their faith.'

The fabric of our professional lives in pathology is woven from the tales of both the living and the dead. Of course, we're always in direct and close touch with our dead, but we're almost always at least one other doctor distant from our living patients. We're used to passing our diagnosis to the clinician and while we never see the patient, we're always aware that there's a real, living person waiting anxiously at the other end for our verdict and to discover their sentence. Our news is often interesting, both to our doctors and to patients.

The Quick and the Dead

Sometimes it's revealing. All too often, it's just devastatingly bad. It's rare that we're able to deliver so clear a reprieve for so obvious a death sentence as I was able to do in Chandra's case.

Yet for doctors of both kinds, all of you, the Quick and the Dead, are our patients and we are privileged to care for you equally.

CHAPTER 1

My Bowels Will Be the Death of Me

'Doctor, there is a three-year-old girl here with much vomiting. I think there is something wrong with her.'

I sighed.

It had been a long day. My wife, Elayne, and I hadn't yet settled down for our evening meal. I was relaxing to the sound and the aroma of chops grilling when the phone rang. It was the surgical ward sister, Dorothy Mombeshora.

'How long has she been vomiting? Is she dehydrated?'

'A few days now, her father says. Before that she was well. But yes, Doctor, she looks dry.'

'Could it be gastroenteritis?' I asked hopefully. In Africa, there is always gastroenteritis around, thanks to the primitive sanitation and the sticky flies that dine in the toilet facilities. If it was just gastro, maybe I could get away with inserting a drip to get her fluids into balance again. Then I could still make it back home in time for the chops.

'No, Doctor. I don't think so. I think she has some trouble in her bowels.'

I trusted Dorothy completely. She had decades of experience, had managed to raise three thriving children of her own, and you couldn't look into her eyes without seeing the steel in her soul. There are many strong women in Africa like that. They have to be.

Bowels in a three-year-old. I racked my brains. What could it be? An intussusception — a painful telescoping of a length of small gut into the next? That was quite common at her age. Perhaps a hernia sac, with trapped bowel stuffed painfully into it?

I sighed again. It could be anything. I would have to go and look.

'I'll be there in five minutes.'

I bade a mental farewell to the chops.

* * *

Precious was a gorgeous little girl. She sat on her mother's lap and looked out at me from huge brown eyes. Her hair was closely plaited and she wore a bright pink dress, white socks and shining, strap-over shoes. She had been dressed in her best to come to see the doctor, as our African patients so often were. Their mothers would sometimes even rub the children's skins with Vaseline jelly to make them look shiny and black and at their best, just so, and to show how much they loved them.

'Well now, little one, what has been happening to you?'

Precious shyly turned her face away into her mother's breast at the sound of my voice. Her father stood behind the chair turning his hat around in his anxious fingers, looking down nervously. I noticed that both parents, the Dambudzos, were dressed in their very best clothes, too.

'Doctor, she will not eat at all.'

Her father looked at me and I could see the pain in his glance. He looked down again. 'Not even ice-cream, which she loves. Doctor, can you cure her? Please?'

I stood up and stepped to the examination bed.

'Let's see what we can do. Please can you undress her and lie her down on the bed here.'

Precious was a gem. She co-operated without a murmur, watching me solemnly as I examined her. I was always impressed by the placid good nature of our African children as patients. I suppose patience and stoicism is handed down from generation to generation in the encounter with the hardships hurled at them by that dangerous continent.

Sister Mombeshora was right. Precious was not well at all. Her temperature was normal but I guessed she was about 5 per cent dehydrated. That much at least I could correct by putting up a drip of half dextrose Darrow's and carefully running in her liquid loss. But what was the cause?

Her little stomach was definitely distended, the skin taut as a drum compared with the dry laxity of the skin around her throat and on her arms. I considered typhoid fever. That caused constipation and vomiting, and the temperature was often normal or low. I felt her stomach carefully, watching her face for pain. And froze.

I could feel a huge mat of tumour encasing the bowels. Cancer! My heart sank. I looked up. Mum and Dad were fearfully watching me. Mr Dambudzo must have seen something in my face. I glimpsed for a second there a look of utmost despair replaced almost as quickly with a look of resignation. I dropped my gaze, embarrassed to have given away so much.

But even as I leapt to it, the conclusion seemed wrong. This didn't really feel like a cancer. This tumour was spread out along the entire colon, feeling more like constipated stools. Other, vaguer lumps were scattered elsewhere in the gut. What the hell could that be? Certainly not any cancer I was aware of.

And then I remembered a lecture delivered one late, drowsy afternoon by the famous parasitologist Professor John Goldsmid, who had made a great name for himself in Africa and then went on to burnish it even more brightly in Tasmania.

Ascaris lumbricoides is a disgusting round worm whose eggs dwell and flourish in moist African soil and go on to infest so many of our children. When an infestation is present in vast numbers, the worms can actually clog up the entire gut. It seems unbelievable, but I had seen buckets and buckets of these revolting writhing worms which had been scooped out by the handful during surgery to clear a bloated and blocked gut.

I knelt beside the bed, my eyes level with Precious's stomach. I had learned you often could actually see these foul worms through the thin skin and stomach wall as they seethed this way and that inside the bowel. I couldn't see any such sinuous slithering, but nevertheless I was convinced this was the right diagnosis. I just knew that my first thoughts of cancer must be wrong. She was far too young, anyway, and far too well nourished to have such a large cancer. Round worms, I thought, for sure.

I explained what I thought to her parents. Precious would need an operation to clear the worms out.

If anything, her father looked even more anguished, having been presented the agony of choice.

'Ah no, Doctor,' he said quietly. 'Please. We do not want an operation. We only want some pills.'

This was a pretty common attitude in Africa. It was widely believed in the bush country that an operation was certain death. It was much better to take your chances with whatever fate or the spirits might grant you. Precious's mother seemed less adamant. She might have been more aware of the gravity of her little daughter's affliction than her husband.

I had in the meantime put up an intravenous drip on Precious, all without a sound or even a grimace from the little patient. She was a true stoic — or perhaps she was just sicker than I thought. I used every shred of persuasion I could on her mum and dad. Sister Mombeshora came and gave me sterling support, forcefully repeating all my arguments in Shona, the language spoken in the area around Gwelo. She was also much louder.

'If we do not operate then I am sorry, but I think Precious might die. There are no pills we know of to help her.'

Finally, the persuasion worked. The father agreed. He was a man in torment, but Precious's mother seemed nothing but relieved.

I phoned the medical superintendent, Gerald Sinclair.

'Gerald, I have a young girl here with intestinal obstruction. I think it may be due to a heavy load of round worms blocking everything up. The X-rays' — I had ordered these in the meantime — 'are odd. Not typical of ascariasis, but I don't know what to make of them. But obstructed for sure and she'll need a laparotomy. Can you come in?'

A three-year-old child would be a complex surgical procedure, well above anything I could ever handle alone, that was for sure. Gerald had done a couple of years as a surgical registrar in Harare Hospital in Salisbury and had a pretty good grounding in the basics of abdominal surgery. I suppose I thought that, between us, we were up to the job in front of us.

Gerald readily agreed and arrived ten minutes later.

He examined Precious and agreed with me that she had a major obstruction. But looking at the X-rays, he shook his head.

'Buggered if I know,' he said, after a long while. 'Looks like ground glass in there to me. Let's open her up. Who's the anaesthetist?'

'Jason.'

Gerald nodded slowly. Jason Moyo was a nurse anaesthetist. Training nurses to fulfil the role of anaesthetist — usually a medical speciality — was a local answer to the disastrous situation we were facing at the time. Rhodesia, soon to become Zimbabwe, was in the throes of a bloody civil war, and was desperately short of doctors of all kinds. Many had already emigrated, while those who remained were called away to serve for months at a time with the colours. I was an Air Force doctor by day, but every afternoon and night I worked as a medical officer in the public hospital. To bridge the ever-widening demand for care, nurses had been intensively trained, initially with some very experienced midwives becoming obstetricians. They were brilliant and soon were successfully carrying out all the ventouse and forceps deliveries formerly done by doctors. The most advanced even learned to do Caesarean sections. This idea was then extended to nurse anaesthetists, and they proved easily capable of anaesthetising our hale and fit young patient population, who had the kind of strong hearts and clean circulations that we in the developed world can only dream of. Soon the nurse anaesthetists were an indispensable part of the surgical team.

Jason had become a very good and experienced anaesthetist. But none of us, doctors or nurse anaesthetists, really knew diddly-squat about operating on paediatric patients. How could we? We had no experience. And there was no-one to teach us.

At first, all went well. Under Jason's care, Precious fell deeply asleep. Jason gave us the nod, and Gerald slit the thin tissue of the midline of the abdominal wall open and the distended bowels burst out of his incision, bloated, purple and wet.

Definitely no cancer there. Thank God for that much, at least. But what was it?

We felt her bowels tentatively between our gloved fingers. The bowels felt heavy. Heavy as lead. Like wheat bags, or draught excluders. Like … like … like something, but we knew not what.

Gerald looked up at me, perplexed. 'Any ideas?'

'Buggered if I know. Doesn't look like ascariasis, that's for sure. This isn't worms.'

'Better open her bowel up and see.'

I lifted the bowel up with one hand while Gerald placed two clamps onto a portion of the wall. I held the clamps up to stop any accidental spillage of faeces into the abdominal cavity as he opened the gut with his scalpel. We looked curiously into the hole.

We stared, dumbfounded. What the hell was that?

Gerald put his finger into the hole and scooped out the contents.

Granular black material came out clumped on the finger of his glove. He held it up to the overhead surgical light. We examined it. He rubbed the tip between his fingers speculatively.

'Sand!' declared Gerald. 'It feels just like bloody sand!'

'Pica!' I breathed out the word. 'My God! It's pica!'

Neither of us had ever seen this before, although we'd heard of it. You couldn't practice in Africa without at least hearing of it. It was often talked about but, in truth, seldom if ever seen by most doctors. Pica is a disorder which consists of literally eating earth. It is not just about a lick or two to get the taste. It's the compulsive eating of prodigious quantities of earth until you're about ready to burst.

Why? Who knew, back then? We thought maybe people were driven to it because of the lack of iron in their diet and the iron deficiency anaemia they got because of this, a theory that seemed to be corroborated by whispers that pregnant women often ate earth.

Of course, the ancient soil of Africa has been endlessly crapped and pissed upon by millions of people for millennia. Because of that constant fouling, it was often full of dormant parasite eggs. Heavy gut infestations of pulsating worms were the usual result. That, of course, just made any blood loss, iron deficiency and anaemia that was already present even worse.

Precious didn't fit this mould at all, though. Why would she be iron deficient? She was well nourished and clearly lived with loving and well-to-do parents. Why in God's name would she eat sand?

That question would have to wait. We still had a job to do. We had to open her bowel and scoop out all this deadly sand that she had swallowed. For no matter why she had done this, it was killing her and it would surely do so unless we unblocked her soon.

We set to work happily. At least we had a practical solution to the problem at hand, scooping out kidney dish after kidney dish of the sticky black sand. It was quite incredible. There were several hundred grams of it and they were solidly blocking segments of her small bowel as well as her colon and rectum. How in the name of God could a three-year-old child have swallowed all this sand, all apparently under the ever-watchful eye of her adoring parents? I just had to wonder.

In the quiet theatre, Gerald and I were making progress. We were milking all the harsh sand through the bowel to the holes we had punctured. We were being very gentle, as we didn't want to pop or even damage the tissue-thin bowel wall with its abrasive contents.

Then there was a susurration from the head of the table. We looked up and met Jason's panicked eyes above the surgical mask he was wearing.

'Something is wrong!' he gasped. 'She has oedema!'

Sure enough, fluid was pouring out of her lungs, clear but frothy. So, so much fluid, I couldn't believe it. This was pulmonary oedema — fluid on the lung — but why?

I looked at the drip. There was a flaccid, empty bag hanging off the stand which should have held the better part of a litre of Ringer's lactate.

'Has she had that entire litre?' I asked, aghast.

Jason stared numbly at the stand for a long moment and nodded.

Oh, God.

Precious was dead. We had killed her.

A whole litre of Ringer's lactate! We had set the wrong flow rate and delivered a massive fluid overload. She had received too much by hundreds of millilitres. We had literally drowned her with our fluid.

It was my fault, I felt — at least, it was our collective fault. We had done our best but it wasn't nearly good enough. While we were absorbed in our strange surgery, we missed the bigger picture and she suffocated in our care.

We did what we could to resuscitate her but it was hopeless. I peeled off my gloves and I trudged slowly out of the operating theatre and down to the ward. It was the hardest journey of my life. The Dambudzos were waiting patiently. They looked up at me, and saw in my face what had happened. They were expecting it, of course: that just made it worse. The Dambudzos deserved better, Precious certainly deserved better, but there was nothing better on offer on that tropical night than our inadequate efforts. I just felt hopeless. What could I say to them?

Mrs Dambudzo started a terrible, keening ululation. Her husband solemnly shook hands with me, and thanked me for all that I had done for his little girl. Only then did he turn to try to comfort his wife. Their reaction will stay with me always. I walked out into the cool evening of the African high veldt. The sky was clear, with the constellations swinging on their ancient way, the hard glitter of the stars reaching me from a billion years ago. It was beautiful, awesome. It was enough to move your soul and make you feel close to God.

'Fuck!' I kicked a dent in my clapped-out car.

Then I crouched by the front wheel and wept.

This was the first and only case of pica I have ever encountered. Apparently it is more complicated than we two inexperienced provincial hospital doctors operating late that night had ever suspected. I found out years later that even today no-one really knows what the hell this disorder is all about.

It is apparently still quite common in Africa, especially during pregnancy and in mothers who lack iron. This, at least, offers a logical explanation: the minimal iron present in the soil may indeed confer some benefit on the eater, but there are other, odder and seemingly related types of eating disorder, too, and they occur right around the world. Some people feel compelled to eat ice, others hair, some glass and — worst of all, as it seems to me — some even eat faeces. All the dogs I have ever owned and yours, too, I am sure, have had the regrettable habit of eating cat poo. It's such a common behaviour that some people call cat faeces 'dog lollies'. Whatever the motivation is for dogs, I suspect it will be quite different from humans who eat faeces. I have to say I am speechless at the thought of humans eating shit. Where do they get it from, for a start?

I have no idea what causes these bizarre behaviours, and I am not alone. Yet they are given official names in Western medicine such as pagophagia for ice, trichophagia for hair and, of course, coprophagia is the unlovely name for eating shit.

I still often think of little Precious and of the dignified Dambudzos. When I do, I am reminded of the words that Oliver Cromwell wrote to his sister and his brother-in-law on the death of their son at the battle of Marston Moor, more than three hundred years before:

'There lies your precious child full of glory, never to know sin or sorrow any more.'

Precious Dambudzo. March 1980. Requiescat in pace.

* * *

'A child is dead at home in Levin and it looks suspicious. Could be another case of child abuse. Would you be able to come and have a look? The CIB are waiting at the scene.'

I groaned inwardly. Not another one!

A high-profile trial had just taken place locally, in which a man had faced criminal charges in relation to the death of an infant who had been brought into hospital dead from a ruptured gut. It was alleged that he — the boyfriend of the victim's mother — had caused the rupture by kicking him in the stomach. The man had been involved in the death in identical circumstances in Hawke's Bay some years before of the child of his previous girlfriend. Back then, in the Bay, his lawyer had managed to convince the court that the child's injuries were due to falling down stairs. It was a preposterous story then, we thought, and it hadn't got any more plausible since.

The book was thrown at him and he was charged with both crimes. Kevin Pringle, a paediatric surgeon, gave evidence, as did I. This time, the jury was in no doubt and he was duly convicted. It was an emotionally draining case: even the successful prosecution didn't feel like a victory. The perpetrator was a damaged soul, and you could argue that he was as much a victim of his tortured personality as either of the infants, with their fragile guts.

And violence against children never seems to come to an end. No sooner have we put one behind us than another case seems to roll on up. This sounded like it might indeed be the next one.

In news stories reporting deaths, you often hear the phrase 'A post-mortem investigation will be carried out tonight'. It sounds routine, but it doesn't do justice to the scale of the task that an autopsy in the mortuary presents, especially if the death is suspicious. Add to that the 40-minute drive south and the same back plus the scene examination, and that was most of my day gone — to say nothing of the many, many hours that would follow if my findings prompted a full-scale homicide investigation.

But I was on call, so there was no ducking it.

'Okay,' I said, taking down the address. 'I'll be there in 40 minutes.'

Imagining the scene that awaited me, my thoughts were dark as I set off. But there's something about the Manawatu countryside — the broad, green plains stretching to the foot of the rugged Tararua Range — that soothes the soul. I was in a much better space by the time I arrived.

The house had seen better days, but it was clean. It was probably a rental, but I guessed the occupiers were good tenants. Shabby was pretty common in the provinces back then, when those at the bottom of the heap were hardest hit by tough economic times. This home was as tidy as could be expected.

I was met at the door by the kind of solid, dispassionate policeman to whom I have become accustomed in my time in the Manawatu. When I asked him what the story was, he just turned back into the house and jerked his head for me to follow. A man of few words, then, like most of them: just ask their wives.

The scene didn't have much to say, either. It was a lounge with a few scattered sticks of chairs and a very weary sofa. There was no reek of old cigarette smoke: there weren't even any ashtrays so far as I could see, and nor was there the scatter of beer bottles common in scenes of domestic dysfunction. Instead, there were toys dotted around the threadbare, greyish carpet, and amongst them, lying cruciform and perfect as a Renaissance painting of Christ on the Cross, there was the body of a child. He was a beautiful blond boy, about four years old, lying flat on his back with his legs straight and his arms flung out at right angles to his body, palms upright. His head was turned gently to the left, chin down, and the only sign that anything was amiss was the small mess of bloody vomit that stained the carpet near his lips. He was pale, abnormally so, and his eyes were becoming milky with the cloudiness of death. His body was uninjured, unbruised, untraumatised, so far as I could see. He was lying completely at peace and I knew at once that he had not been moved since death.

I knelt beside him.

'What has happened to you here, my young fellow?' I murmured to myself, unconsciously paraphrasing the words I had used to Precious all those long years ago.

I looked at the parents. They were huddled at the end of the room clinging to one another for comfort, their younger child enfolded protectively in their arms. To all appearances, they were a pretty average, down-at-heel couple. They looked sorrowful, scared and confused. I sensed that because they had no idea what had happened, they were unsure whether they were to blame.

'Can you tell me what happened?' I asked gently.

'We don't know. It just sort of happened suddenly.'

I didn't have to look at the Criminal Investigation Branch officers to know that their brows were knitted sceptically. Probabilities suggested that this was an assault. Superficially, at least, it didn't look too good for the parents.

'Tell me,' I prompted them quietly.

'He's been a bit grumbly but not bad, so we weren't worried,' his mother said helplessly. 'He didn't seem to be in pain.'

She was mid-twenties, maybe younger. There was no deceit about her that I could see. In fact, if I'd had to describe her, the word 'naïve' would have sprung to mind.

'The kids were playing as usual and then Jack just suddenly vomited, lay down like that as he is there and closed his eyes.'

She began to cry.

'We tried to wake him,' she sobbed, 'but he wouldn't, no matter how hard we tried. I don't know how to do that … thing. You know, that breathing thing for them. We just don't know how.'

Of those of us standing around young Jack's body as it lay on the autopsy table that night — the CIB officers and myself — only I believed her story. The policemen watched as my scalpel split the porcelain perfection of the boy's torso apart and his bowels swelled out for our scrutiny. The cause of death was immediately apparent. There was an unexpected, bright cherry-pink section, about five centimetres long, sitting right in the middle of the small intestine, a beacon that could not help but draw your eye. What was this? It was certainly not the bruised, bleeding, traumatic gut that I was so used to from the assaults inflicted by the 'boyfriend' in the recent criminal case. It was a length of dead and bleeding bowel, but it had suffered from something lurking inside the body, not from a violent attack from outside.

I searched the abdominal cavity. I pushed my gloved fingers deep into the bowl of the pelvis and probed. There was nothing there.

I shook my head.

'What's wrong?' the young detective asked, leaning forward intently. 'What have you found?'

'Nothing,' I replied. 'I was feeling for a femoral hernia sac, thinking the gut may have finished up trapped in a hernia. But there's no hernia there. He's as perfect as the day he was born.'

I couldn't get the image of the young Jesus out of my mind.

'Why isn't it an assault? Like in that last case?' the CIB officer asked.

I shook my head again, puzzled.

'There's no bruising to the abdominal wall or anywhere in the surrounding tissues,' I said, thinking aloud. 'It's definitely not an assault, so it must be natural. But what?'

I knew the CIB needed to be sent home. This was not a job for them.

I felt closely around the mesentery, the fatty flap carrying blood vessels to the gut. Wrapped around it, there was a tight, tough, sinewy band that had captured and constricted the section of bowel to death. This malformation was called a congenital band. Jack would have been born with this python lying in wait in his mesentery. Why it chose that moment after sitting dormant for so many years I can't say, but for Jack, this was his time to die.

'So if that's what killed Jack, why did no-one see he was in distress?' the police asked me. 'Do you reckon this might be negligence? You know, like neglect by the parents?'

'No, I really don't think so,' I replied, then paused to wonder why I could be so certain. 'It's true that it's very odd the parents never saw any signs of a problem. It's not what the books say usually happens. But I am sure they're telling the truth. I suspect no-one would have seen this coming.'

The police were staring at me. I suddenly realised what had convinced me that the parents were telling the truth.

'I mean, you all saw the house there. There were toys scattered on the carpet around him. Those two kids were obviously playing just before it happened, for God's sake! No-one could have set up that family scene so convincingly if they were trying to disguise an assault. Odd as it seems, I reckon Jack was playing happily with his brother all the while he had a bit of dead gut inside of him, and suddenly he rolled over, vomited once and died. Simple as that.'

The cloud of suspicion passed. I could see the policemen nodding in agreement. They had seen the scene for themselves, and it most certainly didn't look like a murder scene. They began packing up the tools of their trade and left the mortuary, gratefully heading for bed. No-one wanted a murder investigation. Tomorrow they would be free for other more important places and jobs.

For me, there was only one mystery remaining. How could such a severe gut problem, which should have been exquisitely painful, have had no visible effect on Jack?

Frankly, I just don't know the answer. We all have differences in our perception of pain or our tolerance of it. Jack must simply have had a very high pain threshold.

I once ruptured an Achilles tendon serving at tennis, at about the same time the All Black Justin Marshall ruptured his just short of the line as a try beckoned. He hopped the last few metres and scored anyway. Opinion was divided on whether he felt the pain of the injury and ignored it long enough to score: I felt nothing at all when I injured mine. This is strange, because the tendon is a highly sensitive organ. I have seen people just about crippled by Achilles tendonitis, a mere swelling of the tendon sheath. Doctors routinely squeeze the Achilles tendon of unconscious patients to test for the sensation of deep pain. Why is pain perception so variable? No-one really knows, but high tolerance for pain must make the diagnosis of many diseases very difficult.

One Sunday morning, a jogger dropped dead not far from my front gate. People tried to revive him but to no avail. He soon arrived at the mortuary, and the autopsy was interesting. My assistant, Bruce Scott, pulled his pluck of organs out of the body cavity, placed the dripping mass in a large bowl in a trolley and wheeled it over.

'There you go, Doc,' he said. 'Ticker job, I reckon.'

If I had a dollar for each time my mortuary assistants had correctly identified the cause of death, I would be a very rich pathologist indeed. It was a 'ticker job': the jogger had suffered a heart attack, that part was easy. I dissected the right coronary artery along its length and an expansive, purplish mass of blood clot oozed out of the vessel. A coronary thrombosis, blocking the blood supply to the posterior part of the left side of the heart. And to confirm this there was an ugly, yellowish-grey discolouration of the heart muscle at precisely the place supplied by that artery.

But the changes in the heart were two weeks old when I examined them under my microscope. How in the hell could he have gone jogging with a two-week-old heart attack? The mystery deepened when I spoke to his wife. She reckoned that for the previous two weeks, he was completely normal: he not only went jogging, he went to work and even had sex on several occasions — all with a severe, advanced heart attack and no hint of discomfort.

I have now seen many times that the silent and completely painless heart attack is a reality, and it is much more common than we realise. But Jack is unique, as his is the only case I have ever come across of silent gut infarction — tissue death — in either adult or child. Whatever caused this to happen without any warning signs did not really matter. Ultimately and tragically, his bowels were to be the death of him.

Jack. 1990. Requiescat in pace.

CHAPTER 2

Troubles with the Liver

The incident happened in the hours of darkness on the ninth night of November 1988, soon after I had arrived in New Zealand.

Our senior general surgeon, John Coutts, turned up just before our mid-morning coffee break the night after the incident. He was still dressed in his scrubs and grinning expansively. He held up a small vial filled with formalin, shook it and said: 'What do you make of these bits of tissue?'

I looked at them. Small, discoloured, brownish-red bits of tissue, but rather necrotic-looking. Pathologically, 'necrotic' means they were dead, broken-down tissue — certainly not what you want in meat you might buy from the butcher.

'Where did you get them from?' I asked cautiously.

John Coutts would only come in in person with something that was a surgical puzzle. He was a hugely experienced and highly competent provincial surgeon, born and bred in Palmerston North, and if he walked down the main street of the city, he would be greeted at every step by folk whose afflicted innards he had exposed to the light of day and surgically corrected over the years.

'Haven't you heard? There was a machine-gun accident up at Waiouru last night.'

I shook my head. There had been nothing in the news that I had heard.

'Where is Waiouru?'

'Ah!' he said, settling back into his characteristic anecdotal mode. 'It's the main New Zealand Army training camp, up on the way to Taupo, before you get to Turangi.' Of course, that left me none the wiser. God only knew where these strange places might be. Elayne and I didn't yet know the country and I was only really certain where Wellington, Auckland and Palmerston North were.

I nodded, all the same.

'The Army had a night-fighting exercise last night. Did you know New Zealanders like night fighting?'

I shook my head again, which was all the encouragement John needed to give me a potted history of New Zealand's nocturnal military accomplishments. It turns out New Zealand soldiers have earned a pretty fierce reputation in the battles of the last century or so and it shows little sign of waning even today. Kiwis seem to prefer to attack during the hours of darkness, and often win the day — or night — due to the sheer bloody shock it gives their enemy. Other, perhaps saner, people look upon night as a time of rest, a time to relax and prepare mentally for the hardships of the day yet to come. Not the Kiwis.

While the Turks and Aussies fought each other to a standstill at Lone Pine on the Gallipoli Peninsula, Brigadier-

General Andrew Russell led his New Zealand mounted regiments in a wild left-hook attack during the depths of the night on a strategically important feature named Chunuk Bair. They captured the heights through a deft combination of skill, daring and guts. As dawn broke, the New Zealanders looked down and saw for the first and last time their ultimate objective, the waters of the Dardanelles Narrows. That glimpse was the closest the ANZACs came to victory. Russell's men were relieved and the relieving force was driven off Chunuk Bair by a Turkish counter-attack. The rest of the campaign is history.

New Zealanders got it done again in a key engagement in the Second World War a little over two and a half decades later. In June 1942, the Kiwis were surrounded by German Field Marshal Rommel's troops at Minqar Qaim in the North African desert. They were expected to surrender at dawn. Instead, they launched an attack just after midnight and bowled through Rommel's positions, leaving him to rue what he called 'gangster fighting methods'.

I was interested to learn all of this. In my experience of African warfare, there wasn't usually much night fighting. Sure, there was the odd night attack, but they were usually half-hearted: the killing really only began at dawn and ended promptly at dusk.

'They had an exercise with live machine-gun firing last night,' John was explaining, getting to the point, 'but it went wrong.'

He grinned happily at me. He was enjoying himself. He had been having surgical fun for sure and I guessed it had gone well. I was beginning to understand the character of the provincial folk amongst whom we had settled.

'The soldiers had to advance rapidly, keeping just behind the machine-gun fire which was marked with tracer rounds so they could track it. They followed the tracer closely and all was going well. Then there was a misfire. The gunner cleared the stoppage and then went on to finish firing the rest of his clip.'

John shook his head, still smiling at me.

'The men were already forward of the line of fire. The rest of the jammed clip was now being fired directly into them.'

No-one had really heard of 'friendly fire' in those days. It would have sounded as absurd to us then as it does now. There's nothing 'friendly' about machine-gun fire, no matter who is subjecting you to it.

As a pathologist, I would have been the first to know about any death, but there hadn't been any bodies in the mortuary that morning.

'What happened to them?' I asked.

'It was 3.30 a.m. The medic of the section was Sergeant Jon Brausch. Amazingly, he was the only one hit but he took it hard. He was hit by eight separate bullets. The other soldiers did a pretty good job of putting on field dressings and in 20 minutes a medic arrived just as he was losing consciousness.'

Most people have heard of the so-called Golden Hour — the critical period immediately following major trauma when medical attention has the highest likelihood of preventing death. It is said to have first been recognised on the grim battlefields of Flanders and France back in the First World War. The concept has since caught people's imaginations, although medical and surgical experts in critical care are sceptical, with some going so far as to call the Golden Hour an urban myth. Modern medical literature apparently holds that there is no 'magic' period of time. The quicker the better for sure, that goes without saying, but statistically, the Golden Hour doesn't exist. Be that as it may, the idea is part of our belief system and we are all very happy to have the rescue helicopter standing by to bring the casualties in from the roads, the mountains and the forests just as fast as they can. And if they can do it inside that Golden Hour, surely that has to be a good thing?

'The army medics got two drips up and two litres of Haemaccel into him,' John said. I grimaced at that. I had personally never used Haemaccel — a colloidal solution containing rendered-down gelatin that was supposed to serve as a 'volumiser' to keep blood pressure from falling dangerously low. Some doctors swear by it. We were told in Africa that it was okay for vets to use on dogs but better to stick to Ringer's lactate for people.

'They placed him in mast pressure pants, wrapped him in a gold-leaf blanket for warmth and were lucky enough to get the rescue helicopter from Taupo to the scene. He got here at 5.30 a.m., we topped him up with some blood and he was in theatre by six.'

The way into Palmerston North was clagged in with cloud. The weather was clear to Taupo but the hospital there couldn't have handled such severe injuries. Fortunately for the wounded soldier, the Taupo rescue helicopter had recently been set up with night-vision gear — the first in the country to be so equipped — and the pilot, John Funnell, decided to have a go at getting into Palmerston North. Through skill and guts, he succeeded. It meant that Brausch was lying on the operating table in theatre just two and a half hours after the first bullet struck him. That could only have been bettered if there had already been a helicopter with night-flying capability standing by at Waiouru in the wee hours. The closest Air Force helicopter was at Ohakea, and it wasn't even on standby to scramble.

'Eight hits? That sounds as if it should have been instantly fatal. I've never seen anyone survive anything like that number of hits. What did you find?'

'A big hole blown in the chest wall. It chipped off splinters of rib and there were fragments of muscle around that were dark and felt like papier mâché. They weren't contracting so I decided they were dead. I scraped and debrided those out until it all looked clean and healthy.'

He paused. 'There was also a 15-centimetre hole in the lumbar region of the back. The bleeding from that round reached right into the fat around the kidney, but the kidney itself was okay. But this hit caused another problem.'

John stopped for a moment and leaned forward, picking up the vial containing the tissue from where it sat on the table. He tapped it on the tabletop, making the fragments swirl and dance.

'These I found floating freely in blood lying in the abdomen. The cavity was full of blood and air and there was bruising to the bowel. But what are these bits?'

I took the vial and examined them closely.

'Liver?' I guessed.

John nodded happily at me. 'Yes, that's what I thought! It's odd, because the bullet track was well clear of the liver. But a four-centimetre swathe of the liver itself was macerated and crumbly, so my guess is that these are bits of liver. Can you have a look and confirm it?'

I nodded.

I heard how Jon Brausch also had slashing wounds to the rim of the pelvis, the buttocks, the thigh and the knee. He was lucky in so many ways, quite apart from the speed of his casevac from the training area and into the hands of a highly competent surgeon.

His liver tissue was fascinating. I examined his slides under the microscope a few days later. There were ugly, irregularly shaped zones of devitalised, necrotic tissue ending at an uneven but distinct border with healthy normal liver. This was an odd pattern of damage that I had never seen before.

My mind churned through the possibilities.

Zones of liver-cell death or necrosis, as we call it, are a favourite pattern-recognition game for young pathologists to play. For example, in the simple lobule of the liver, cells around the portals carrying the bile ducts and blood vessels to and from the gut always die first in poisonings such as in suicides from paracetamol overdose. After the substance has been absorbed from the gut, the first place it unloads its burden of toxins is in that zone — the 'peri-portal zone' — of the liver.

You see the same effect in cases of accidental phosphorus poisoning. It's ancient history now, but the women and children in the factories who used to make phosphorus-based 'safety' matches in our great-grandparents' day died in droves as the poisonous element rotted the peri-portal zones of their livers. It also caused their jawbones to collapse grotesquely into a mushy soup. That's progress for you: who knows how many were spared death by burning from the unpredictable wax matches that preceded 'safety' matches?

The very innermost zone of liver closest to the veins dies in carbon tetrachloride poisoning. Who might get that?

Apparently the dry-cleaners of clothes used to. The middle zone between these two zones characteristically becomes necrotic in yellow fever, but you need to be in West Africa or South America to get that. Poisonous mushrooms attack all three zones without apparent discrimination.

Jon Brausch's liver death was untidily random, fitting none of the established patterns, which were obviously irrelevant anyway, given that it arose from a gunshot injury rather than poisoning.

I told John Coutts what I had found and described the strange pattern of necrosis.

'I can only think that this must be the distant effect of the advancing supersonic shock wave from the bullet. It must be a pretty high-velocity bullet to do that amount of damage without actually hitting the liver.'

John had confirmed that there was no direct hit by the bullet on the liver, but John being John, he had since found out all about the weapon involved. He loved weapons. He had a pretty good collection and an encyclopaedic knowledge of weapons quite apart from the ones he owned.

'It was a light machine gun called a C9 Minimi which fires 1100 5.56-millimetre-calibre rounds a minute.'

'Pretty small projectile,' I said. 'The old FN rifles in Africa used 7.62-millimetre rounds.'

'Yes, but it's very high velocity!' John's eyes glistened with excitement. 'Its muzzle velocity is 3200 feet per second!'

I was impressed and appalled at the same time. Setting aside the morality of it, the calculation that arms manufacturers use in designing their wares is quite simple. In order to rip apart the human body, it's just like a traffic accident, really — it's exactly as the road safety slogan warns us: 'The faster you go, the bigger the mess.' Soldiers, of course, take a humorous view of it all:

In any conflict some may fall
Let's hope that we're not shot at all
But if it happens that we are hit
Let's hope it's not a vital bit
And most of all if shot we be
It's not at high velocity.

But 3200 feet per second is fast, very fast. The crateriform FN rifle injuries I saw in Africa were inflicted by heavier bullets but with a velocity of only 2800 feet per second. Each of the rounds that had ploughed into Jon Brausch did so with nearly 15 per cent more hitting power. How could anyone survive that?

'It must have been the supersonic wave in front of the bullet that did this to his liver,' I repeated to John several months later when he dropped in to give a progress report on how well Jon had recovered.

He shook his head and flashed me that trademark grin.

'That's what I used to think too, but it's not so. I wrote to Colonel Martin L. Fackler, who is the director of the Wound Ballistics Laboratory, about Jon's case. He's at the Letterman Army Institute of Research in San Francisco. He knows a thing or two. He was a surgeon in the thick of the fighting in Da Nang back in the '60s, so he's seen the real stuff. He's done all sorts of experiments firing different types of rifles and ammo at gelatin blocks as well as at pigs.'

John then drew me a diagram to show what happens when a high-velocity round tears into your body.

Troubles with the Liver

'The supersonic wave in front is at its strongest as it punches through your skin and that causes a hole, but the energy is quickly bled away into the local tissue and doesn't do any more harm deeper in. And as we now know, the supersonic waves are not really all that harmful to soft tissue. I mean, we use the same waves to smash kidney stones in the lithotripter, don't we?'

I thought about that for a moment. It was true. The renal lithotripter was a great, power-guzzling electromagnet that pulverised kidney stones with its sonic waves. It bruised the surrounding soft tissue, so that people who have been battered by this treatment walk hunched over as if they have had the shit kicked out of them for a few days. But they soon get better. They are certainly much better off than they would be if they'd gone under the knife and had their muscles and nerves cut through and permanently scarred.

'Anyway, Martin Fackler's shown our old ideas were quite wrong. The bullet drags a big soap bubble about 15 centimetres across behind it, and not in front of it as we'd all believed. This bubble is very much bigger than we realised, and it stretches the tissues to buggery for that whole 15 centimetres, ripping them away from their blood vessels. Then it just pops. It's the bubble behind that does the damage. Solid, inelastic liver does really badly, apparently. It just bursts, loses its blood supply and is polished off pretty quickly.'

I nodded, fascinated. It made sense, and it also explained where those free-floating fragments of dead liver rattling around in Jon Brausch's abdominal cavity came from. To see just how devastating this effect can be, measure out 15 centimetres anywhere on your body.

'The bubble collapses down in milliseconds, leaving a permanent, small, bullet-sized track through the body. Traditionally, we thought that's where all the tissue damage is.'

We pathologists know that 'permanent' track very well indeed. It seems really narrow but is plugged full with cooked blood and dead, pulped tissue. We pass metal probes into the wounds to discover the angle and direction the bullet took so we can piece together just what happened so as to, say, distinguish a suicide from a murder. What John was telling me meant that the inexperienced young surgeon may neatly clean out the narrow track that he can see and never even realise that the dead tissue stretches for another five or six centimetres all around it. Left alone, this necrotic tissue will surely become purulent and quite likely kill the victim. Similarly, as the case of Jon's liver had demonstrated, damage to distant and apparently uninvolved organs is also possible, which is why a gunshot patient may sink despite clever surgery to their obvious wounds.

Jon Brausch had a bit of a rocky recovery with a couple of clean-up operations needed and another peek inside his abdomen to make sure no further mischief was brewing unseen within. These were minor setbacks in the scheme of things. He had youth, fitness and resilience on his side, and 15 days after being hit, he was well on the mend. He told me that when hit, he had made a conscious decision to live. He reckons that it was mind over matter as much as anything else that kept him going until help came.

That is a story that comes up endlessly: the sheer determination to live, to hold on against the odds. There's often also a determination to live well afterwards. You'll see it in the cases of many of those whose stories are told in this book.

Troubles with the Liver

Thank God for John Coutts, surgeon extraordinaire. Thank God, too, for one of the greatest-ever rescue pilots, John Funnell. And thank God for Jon Brausch's sheer will to survive. Valete! We salute you all!

* * *

Jon Brausch was not the first such military high-velocity gunshot injury I had seen, although what I learned from his case finally explained some things I had seen in Africa.

Ten years before, in October 1978, the Rhodesian war was reaching a crescendo. I was in the Zambezi Valley, the hottest part of the country at the hottest time of the year: not for nothing was this called the 'Suicide Month'. Needless to say, I wasn't there by choice. I was the sole medical officer based at the airfield in Kariba, providing cover for about two dozen SAS troopers and a single Lynx light ground attack aircraft to support their operations.

A photo reconnaissance flight had indicated a highly camouflaged encampment with impressive anti-aircraft defences hard by the border on the northern bank of the Zambezi River. The intelligence suggested there was a Russian-trained battalion of some 800 men preparing to launch a conventional assault on Kariba, the town that had grown up around Kariba Dam and its power station. This dam was the major supplier of electricity in central Africa and would be a prime prize to capture.

On the day in question, dinner at the airfield was almost ready — steaks, half an inch thick, and chips. I was happily readying myself to tackle that lot when an airman came up to me.

'Doc, the CO wants you now.'

The other ranks were pretty casual with us doctors. They knew we weren't real soldiers.

I ran over to the command centre, where there were several officers gathered around the CO. He was a squadron leader, soon to be replaced by a group captain as the scale of the imminent enemy operation became apparent.

'We have a request for casevac,' the CO barked. 'You have to go right now!'

My stomach churned. The adrenal glands in my lower back pumped raw adrenaline into my system, preparing me for flight or fight. Which was it to be this time? Perhaps both?

'What's the task?' I asked. Whatever it was, it wouldn't be good at this time of night.

He opened his mouth to answer, but one of the other officers tapped him on the shoulder.

'Wait a minute!' the CO said to me irritably, raising his hand to hold me there. The officer spoke urgently into his ear. He listened, nodded and turned back to me.

'It's all off!' He wiped both his hands horizontally in the washout gesture.

As a lowly flight lieutenant, I knew better than to ask for an explanation. I found out the facts shortly afterwards, sitting next to one of the chopper pilots as we ate dinner in the makeshift messroom.

'There is a ridge running through the middle of the enemy camp,' he told me, chewing on his steak. 'We dropped two groups of the SAS, one on either side. They wormed their way up during the day but at last light they came under fire from the enemy. One bloke hit. Needs evacuation right now but,' he turned and gestured at the clear, star-studded sky, 'it's already too dark to find them in the bush. That's why it was washed out. But we're going in to get him at dawn tomorrow. Should be interesting.'

It was news to me that I would be going in the next day. The adrenaline, which had more or less faded from my bloodstream, came surging back.

'You going to eat that?' the pilot asked, noticing the way I was looking at my steak.

I was up and ready by 0400, long before dawn. I had checked and rechecked my pack: three litres of Ringer's lactate, intravenous needles, pressure bandages, a chest drain, laryngoscope and endotracheal tubes, a tracheostomy set, morphine and intravenous Flagyl to run in for gut wounds. Everything I needed for most eventualities was there. What more could I possibly need, besides a hundred years' experience rather than just the one, and perhaps a big, fully staffed hospital to back me up?

I shivered as I waited, but it wasn't cold. The air was still cloyingly hot although its fierce edge had been radiated off up into the night towards the dome of sentinel stars.

I made my way out to the helicopter, a big, heavy Bell 205 — the same workhorse known as the Huey Cobra to the Americans in Vietnam, but a Cheetah to us. Why this great, loud, cumbersome machine was named for the fast, sleek, silent African cat was a mystery to me, but I wasted no time on it. I climbed aboard and seated myself on the hard bench in the back, my pack by my feet. The pilot and tech-gunner tramped up out of the night and began their pre-flight preparations. The pilot in his helmet and heavy flak vest climbed into his seat and soon lights began to flicker on and instruments to quietly whirr. The gunner walked around the machine and then, pre-flight checks finished, clambered aboard and began arming his twin Browning machine guns. I felt suddenly sick so I leapt out, ran to the back of the chopper and vomited onto the grass of the airfield. That helped. I stood and urinated, looking up at the stars. Briefly and faintly on a light breeze the swampy aroma of the distant lake wafted over us. Then the wind dropped, and it was replaced by the ugly, acrid smell of urine and vomit rising in equal measure from beneath my feet.

'Ready, Doc?' the gunner called back to me, grinning.

I nodded and climbed back aboard. We heaved off the ground and swung away north towards our objective.

It was a beautiful flight.

We flew cloaked in darkness over Lake Kariba towards the Zambian hills, hunched low in the distance like a herd of grazing dinosaurs. That's where my wounded casevac was waiting for me — and where the enemy were. Away in the east, there was a tinge of pink, the merest touch of light on the horizon. That had to be the dawn.

The speed of the machine rammed air cooled by the vast lake below through the open doors of the helicopter. I was cold, yet I was also entranced by the vista. Then, suddenly and unexpectedly, the air sweeping inwards grew hot again as we passed over the northern shoreline and found ourselves back over land. The gunner was extra alert now and swung his barrels this way and that in anxious, small arcs, peering over his sights.

Anytime now.

We dropped abruptly into the bush, the huge blades just clearing the canopy, and touched lightly to the ground.

I looked around. Scraggly grass, scattered clumps of low bushes and darker, taller encircling trees were all that I could see through the maelstrom of dust and debris kicked up by the rotors. It was quite deserted. Extraordinary. What was I to do? Where was I to go?

Then, out of the shrubs no more than three metres from the door of the helicopter, four SAS troopers rose out of the invisibility, their faces streaked with camouflage paint. They ran forward and hurled something heavy at my feet. And just as suddenly, they were gone, invisible once more.

I looked down. The object they had delivered was a body, that of Lance-Corporal John McLauren of C Squadron, the SAS Regiment. He had died in the night five hours after being hit, without medical help and deep inside enemy territory. But he was never alone. His mates lay on guard keeping him company as he faded away.

Instead of medics, Haemaccel and a Golden Hour casevac into the care of a competent surgeon in a modern hospital, John McLauren had only me, woefully inexperienced and arriving well after the fact. I sat with the boy at my feet as the Bell chuntered back across the huge lake into the polished face of a sunrise of gold. The base medics were waiting ready with their kit and skills, raring to do whatever it took to relay this wounded soldier on to help and safety. But as I climbed out, keeping low beneath the hiss of the rotors, I gave the washout sign to them. Their shoulders slumped as they turned away, resigned to another unaffordable tragedy. We had too many of those.

Later, I drove John McLauren's body up to the hospital in the medics' rattly old Land Rover. The state of Rhodesia was on the point of collapse, but I still had an autopsy to do, and a report to file for the magistrate who was acting as coroner. The civil war had been raging for ten years, but John McLauren's death was still regarded as an unnatural death by the civil authorities. It had to be fully investigated and reported.

Diederik van Zyl was the government medical officer in charge at Kariba Hospital. He limped up to the gurney in the primitive, corrugated-iron hut that served as a mortuary. He had told me he had a Perthes hip, where he had slipped something in his joint while a teenager. Ever since, he had walked with a limp. This had excused him from military service, but it didn't stop him doing his bit in the hospital. He was a fine doctor.

The temperature inside the mortuary must have been 50 degrees. It stank foully. Neither the heat nor the smell seemed to bother Diederik, who picked up a scalpel and split John McLauren's stomach open with a brisk slash. The bowels spilled out, pink and yellow, looking healthy enough. But wait. Bloody fluid trickled out, followed by clots of blood that fell with a liquid plop on the concrete floor like a kilogram of raw steak. The clots bounced and blood splashed over the 'veldtschoens' — the rough buckhide shoes we all wore — and up over our bare legs. Neither of us so much as blinked.

We were minimally clad in camouflage shorts and T-shirts, with a token rubber apron that had been roughly hosed down after the last autopsy by the mortuary man. Hygienically, it was all a far cry from the double-gowned, face-masked, rubber-booted, double-gloved autopsies in our spotless mortuaries of today. Health and safety officers would have had conniptions, but it was all just a reflection of the realities. We were accustomed to working daily on wards packed with patients, sharing their breath and their dangers even as we cared for them. Some had open tuberculosis, desperately hacking out their rotted lungs into sputum mugs, like ripe Camembert tinged with bright, fresh blood. Others had meningococcal meningitis, infectious and deadly. Some even frothed with the spume of advanced rabies, which was 100 per cent fatal: we had to tie those tragic cases to their beds, both for our other patients' safety and for our own. All of this was just part of being a doctor in Africa.

There may be doctors and nurses who recall the tuberculosis hospitals in Waipukurau and other centres, where conditions may have been something like what we faced on a daily basis in Africa, but those memories are fading fast. As someone once put it, we don't know how lucky we are these days.

'Lots of free blood in the abdomen. Looks like he's bled out from the gut,' I said.

That is what we had expected to find.

'Ja,' said Diederik. 'Looks like it.' But then he shook his head. He pulled the loops of gut out hand over hand and bent over, peering at the fatty mesentery and the blood vessels attached across the spine. 'No, man. Bowel's intact. No injury here. No bleeding.'

We weren't pathologists, of course. We were just two young boys recently out of medical school, playing at being specialists because there was no alternative. We returned to the path of the bullet, which had entered John's right side, travelled across his abdomen and exited through his left side. We thought he was probably moving forward when he was struck by unexpected flanking fire from the right. That's exactly what the other members of his squad told us later. He only took one hit, but one hit was all it took.

'It's gone right through his liver, clean as a whistle,' I said. I pulled the right lobe of the liver up to see where the bullet had come out of that organ just above the stomach. The left side of the abdomen had been extensively damaged by that bubble that the bullet would have dragged, but miraculously, although it had started tumbling end over end after passing through the liver, it hadn't directly struck anything else vital. God only knows what else we probably missed, but to our inexperienced eyes, the perforation of the liver seemed to be the only injury.

There was a large, star-shaped wound in the left flank where the tumbling bullet had torn its way out.

Diederik and I looked at each other.

'Crap!' I said. 'That's all he had. He's bled out from his liver.'

Diederik nodded. 'Looks like it.'

Yet there was something odd here. In other cases I had seen, there were always huge cavities at the entry point that caused instant death. But in this case, the track through the liver was pretty clean. The bullet had punched straight through without the usual, horrific pulping of tissue. The worst feature of John McLauren's wound was that it looked to me as though it would have been survivable if we'd been able to get him out. His single wound looked a much, much better bet than those hits that Jon Brausch took all those years later.

So what had happened here? He had lived a full five hours after being hit in the liver by a very high-velocity military round. The injury can't have been too bad, much as we'd figured. The real question was why wasn't John McLauren killed instantly, as logic said he should have been?

Troubles with the Liver

As I compared notes with other doctors in subsequent months, I learned that gunshot injuries sustained on our northern border often seemed a bit less severe. Everyone was using the same AK-47 rifle. I couldn't see a reason for the difference, at the time: all I knew was that our northern adversaries were Russian trained and armed, while those on the eastern border were trained and equipped by North Korea, China and, importantly, Yugoslavia.

It was three decades later, when researching the characteristics of Jon Brausch's injuries, that I learned that the Russian ammunition supplied to the ZIPRA Army on the Zambezi was quite different from the Yugoslav rounds supplied to the ZANLA guerrillas in Mozambique. Both types of bullet left the rifle with a muzzle velocity of only 2340 feet per second, which gave them 40 per cent less hitting power than the ammunition used in the NATO FN rifles used by the Rhodesian Army. But the two nations' bullets behave very differently once they hit you, according to the knowledgeable Colonel Fackler. The Russian bullet travels with its point straight forward, and doesn't inflict any significant destruction for about 26 centimetres. Only then does it begin to tumble, which is when it blows up and pops up its devastating bubble. It was just such a projectile that passed pretty cleanly through John McLauren's liver, only blowing a destructive bubble on the other side. The Yugoslav bullet is quite different. It starts tumbling very soon after impact, and typically destroys three times the amount of tissue.

Why, I wondered, would the Russians create a bullet for a military rifle that would inflict much less destruction? Surely they had their own experts equivalent to Colonel Martin Fackler, in which case this must be deliberately designed?

The Quick and the Dead

Apparently, that's exactly what it was. It's the singularly deadly calculation of the arms manufacturer again. The Russian idea was not to kill outright: the dead are cheap and easy to bury, after all. Better to overload enemy medical resources with casualties. It's the same thinking behind anti-personnel mines, which are designed to maim terribly rather than kill: create casualties, a heavy hospital burden and assault civilian morale.

Thanks to some weapon designer's grasp of physics, the injury that John McLauren sustained was survivable. But all of it was irrelevant, really. The stars still wheeled above in the clear tropical sky, marking the passing of the Golden Hour and four more besides and it was all too late.

As the stars that shall be bright when we are dust,
Moving in marches upon the heavenly plain,
As the stars that are starry in the time of our darkness,
To the end, to the end, they remain.
—Laurence Binyon, 'For the Fallen' (September 1914)

The saving of Jon Brausch is a tribute to his care and especially to John Coutts, Surgeon. Would that things had been different for you, John McLauren.

Lance-Corporal John McLauren, C Squadron, SAS.
October 1978. Requiescat in pace.

CHAPTER 3

The Creatures Within Us

'Any idea what this is?' Bruce Lockett waved a specimen container in front of me. 'The GP cut it out as an ordinary sebaceous cyst of the scalp from one of his patients.'

I studied the container. Inside was a creamy-coloured, segmented grub, the shape of a lightbulb with a small black cap at one end. I recognised it immediately, and had to suppress the urge to recoil.

'That's a putzi fly grub! I last saw one of those 40 years ago.'

'Putzi fly? What the hell is that?'

My mind flicked back to the early winter of 1967. I was 13 years old and swaggering around in my newly washed rugby jersey. During my very first practice game for the season, I was roughly grabbed around the neck in a maul and squeezed by my team mate. I felt two or three stabs of pain at the base of my neck and the discomfort persisted throughout the game. Afterwards, in the shower, I could see two red spots on my skin.

Pimples, I thought, and put them out of my mind. Most of us were throwing up our first experimental pimples as we stumbled into puberty.

But these pimples did not run true to form. They grew and grew, until they were embarrassing. I covered them with plasters and told no-one. They weren't painful or even itchy but I kept getting this strange feeling that something wasn't right. In fact, I got the distinct feeling that something was moving in there.

One day, when everyone in the family was out, I carefully locked the bathroom door and closely examined the lumps in my father's magnified shaving mirror. And suddenly I saw they were indeed moving up and down. A small, dark periscope was pumping up and down out through my skin at the head of each pimple. I watched with horror and disgust. When I touched it, the periscope vanished inside of me and became still. After a bit, it cautiously popped out again, made a few exploratory wriggles and then happily began its pistoning in and out again.

I was appalled and mortified at the same time. It was another week before I told anyone. Finally I confided in my older brother, Lawrence. He knew all about animals, kept snakes and had a harrier hawk as a semi-tame pet. He would know what to do.

My worst fears were confirmed as he looked, grimaced and then retched. He stood there staring at me, wiping his mouth with the back of his hand.

'Aggh, *sies* man!' He used the Southern African slang used for anything that was revolting. 'You're just bloody disgusting. It's a *gogo*! Where the hell did you get it from?'

Gogo was local slang for an insect.

I wept a little then. I just couldn't help it. Where would it end?

Lawrence had no idea what it was. I made him swear not to tell anybody. He readily agreed, and the look of utter revulsion as he did so made me wonder if I'd been wise in telling him about it at all.

Soon afterwards, my sharp-eyed grandmother spotted the plasters as we were getting up from the breakfast table.

'What are those plasters covering?' she demanded, and when I did not answer she suddenly grabbed me, pulled me towards her and tore the plaster away. She bent over, peered intently at my shame and then gasped in disbelief. Her eyes became steely.

'Joan! Joan!' She summoned my mother. 'Look at this!'

She spun me around and wrenched my head down to one side to bare my neck as if for an execution. I will never forget her words.

'This boy is riddled with putzi flies!' she crowed. 'I've told you and told you the servants aren't ironing the washing properly!'

My grandmother had been waging a long-standing campaign to assume suzerainty over the family home and give orders to our cook and gardener. My itchy lumps were further ammunition in her relentless struggle.

Putzi flies. The name still makes me shudder half a century later.

I was taken to our GP, Dr O'Brien, an urgent appointment. He examined me, and then sent me out of the room. I wasn't party to the discussion that followed: this was standard in those days. My father explained it all gently to me that night.

'The flies lay their eggs, which hatch into grubs called larvae. They have sharp fangs with which they bite a hole in your skin and crawl inside. The skin closes over except for a breathing hole and they grow and grow inside their little cave.'

'What happens to them? Will they be there forever?'

It was so awful. As if adolescence wasn't enough, I had these things writhing inside me — three of the little monsters in my body, all around my neck just like old-fashioned collar studs. I was terrified that I would carry these creatures with me for the rest of my life. I think I was psychologically scarred: years later, I was traumatised all over again as I watched the movie *Alien*, where a creature erupts from the ribcage of a man in whose chest it has been pupating. That was exactly how I imagined these ghastly grubs.

My dad tried to reassure me.

'They will eventually hatch and a fly will climb out and go. It will be all right in time.'

I couldn't see *that* being all right at all! God, I could just imagine a fly wet and dripping like a baby crawling out of my neck in front of everyone as we sat in Mrs Chambers' Latin or Mr Conchar's History lesson. My life would be over. I would be 'Fly Boy' forever. My. Life. Was. Over.

'Why can't Dr O'Brien take them out?'

'He says he can write a note to a surgeon to ask him to cut them out but that will mean an anaesthetic and an operation. And there could be infection. He thinks we should just let nature take its course.'

In desperation, I went to my grandmother. This time I was weeping properly.

'You have to do something!' I wailed. 'You have to get them out!'

'Be quiet, boy!' she snapped. 'I will get them out. But stop blubbing! It doesn't help, you know.'

I stopped and looked up hopefully, wiping my nose on the back of my sleeve.

'Don't be disgusting! Here's a tissue!'

She was as tough as an old boot, my grandma Maude. The men who courted her as a young girl mostly fell on the Somme at Delville Wood, and her husband, my grandfather, finally died the year I was born of the diseases and injuries sustained fighting in German East Africa. She carried a sadness within her, but hid it well. All the same, the look that she was giving me was kindly and reassuring. Maude was always medically very sure of herself. I felt some hope at last.

'Now tell me: when did it start? How did you notice it?'

I explained about the rugby practice.

'Ja, I remember!' she said, her eyes gleaming. 'That's when it must have happened. You needed the jersey for Monday-afternoon practice, but you only put it in the wash on Sunday night. Naison washed it on Monday morning and ironed it before lunch to be ready for you. But it was still damp and he didn't iron the collar properly. There is where your putzi flies have come from!'

'What do you mean?'

'The flies lay their eggs into wet washing and they hatch out in an hour or two. I tell the servants over and over to dry the washing properly and then iron it with a very hot iron to kill the eggs and the grubs. But because they can't see them, they don't believe me, and your mother thinks I'm a foolish old woman, too. But that is also why we iron all our sheets too. The British laugh at us and say we colonialists want to iron the creases out of our sheets and pillow cases just to show we have servants. But it's not true!' She beat her fist on her breast. 'I would gladly iron them all myself just to keep the putzi flies away! It's your rugby jersey that was the culprit! Those servants!' she tutted to herself.

'But how do I get the maggots out?' I felt like crying again, but I didn't dare. 'I hate them!'

'Ach, they're disgusting,' she agreed. 'But I can help you.'

Grandma Maude was gone a while and then came back to her room with a sharp knife and a plate containing a fat, raw rasher of bacon. I watched apprehensively.

'Are you going to cut them out?' That idea didn't appeal at all, but knowing my grandma, it had to be a distinct possibility.

'No, you stupid boy! Just sit there and be still now.'

I watched as she cut three squares of thick, white bacon fat, each one centimetre by one centimetre. One by one, she carefully placed the bacon fat over the maggots' breathing holes and secured each in place with a large swatch of tough, pink surgical plaster.

'There.' She patted the last one on the back of my neck with satisfaction. 'That'll fix you, you *skelm*!'

A *skelm* was a bad insect or animal or sometimes a bad man in Africa. It was appropriate: I was part insect and part bad boy at that moment.

'What have you done? Are they gone?'

'No, boy. Now you must wait.'

The young have no patience and I had no insight.

'How long? I hate them!' I was wondering whether to indulge myself in tears again. 'Why aren't they gone now?'

Grandma smiled kindly at me and patted the side of her bed. 'Come and sit and I will explain what we are going to do.' I sat next to her and she put her arm around me. 'We are going to fish those *skelm* maggots out. They are finished already. You see, they can't breathe through the bacon fat so they have to make their breathing hole longer until they reach the air at the top of the bacon. That they will do easily enough. Then they will put up their breathing tube to drink in the fresh air they need and what will happen?'

Maude chuckled in expectation.

'I will tell you. Their breathing tubes will stick to the plasters so that they can't go back down into their caves. When the time is ripe, we'll pull off the plasters and the whole lot — lock, stock and maggots — will come out, still stuck to the plaster! The maggot's body will come easily because he will already be halfway out of his cave in the bacon fat just to reach the air to breathe!'

Eight hours later, at dawn, I went and woke my grandma. She ripped the plasters off and grotesquely hanging stuck to each of the adhesive sides were the plump, segmented, pulsating maggots. I will never until the day I die forget the horrible sight of them, plucked ripe from my body. I remember that the maggots' warbles, which are what the caves in my skin were called, were gone by the next day. A minor red spot was all that remained of those awful aliens.

My grandma Maude sure knew a thing or two that my doctor didn't.

The beast that Bruce Lockett waved before me could have been an identical twin to any of the three, loathsome beasts that dangled from those plasters half a century before.

I told Bruce all about the putzi fly and my personal experience of its horrible habits.

'I suppose this is a patient recently back from Africa?' I queried. 'We called it putzi fly, but in much of Africa, it's called tumbu disease. Apparently it's very common, although the only case I ever saw was my own!'

Bruce went to inquire.

'Not from Africa, after all,' he said, after consulting the patient's GP. 'He's a Kiwi.'

I looked up in surprise. 'Really? So where'd he get it?'

'Brazil. He's just back from the Amazon. I've looked it up. It's basically the same, but they call it *hura* in Brazil. Same sort of fly, same basic mechanism, but this one has a clever variation on your African one.'

'What's that?'

'It seems unbelievable, but the female fly grabs a female mosquito and attaches her eggs to the mosquito's abdomen. When the mosquito bites someone, the fly's larvae falls onto the skin and crawls into the hole the bite has made. There it grows into the maggot.'

'Incredible. I guess even my grandma couldn't have blamed the servants for that.'

Since then, I have seen a specimen of the brain of an infant from Panama who died from malaria, which is common there. As an unexpected finding, she had several warbles in the scalp and one which had been bored through the anterior fontanelle, the soft spot that persists in the skull of a newborn until fusion of the bone plates occurs. The warble and maggot lay grotesquely nestled within the brain itself.

That poor child must have suffered hugely. My affliction, so dreadful for a 13-year-old, paled in comparison.

* * *

We don't, thank God, have putzi flies in New Zealand. We live in a temperate paradise, really, and give or take a little giardia, we are relatively free from the hordes of loathsome parasites infesting the warm and wet parts of the globe. Yet we have to keep a constant vigil for people who travel abroad and return or who migrate and bring them to our medical doorstep.

'Can you look urgently at a woman's colon biopsies for me?'

Ross Hayton is a jovial, bearded physician who has done so many colonoscopies in his life that if the lengths of bowel he had inspected were laid end to end, the glistening, pink tube would easily stretch around the planet. Maybe even more than once. I often wondered how he kept his unflagging good humour despite day after day spent stooped and peering down the endoscope deeply embedded in a procession of strange backsides. When he came to see us, it must have been a relief to look someone in the eye for a change.

'Sure.' I looked up from my microscope. 'What's her story?'

'Achara Nok is in a bad way. I don't think she'll pull through this one. She got really bad vasculitis and I reckon it's now affected her bowel.'

'Nasty,' I replied.

Vasculitis is a kind of body's own goal, where your immune system attacks and destroys your own blood vessels. It is often fatal unless the fires of inflammation can be quenched with drugs and the blood vessels saved.

'What treatment is she on?'

'The maximum. High-dose steroids and cyclophosphamide. Not touching it, though. Her diarrhoea has become bloody and it's getting worse, if anything. I thought you could look at these,' he waved a plastic biohazard bag in which there were three pottles holding nubbins of bloody tissue, 'and see if you can spot the vasculitis. Though what more we can do to turn it off, I'm buggered if I know.'

The specimens were rushed through processing in the lab and I had the slides early the next morning. A diagnosis was elusive. There was blood and pus and damaged tissue, but no obvious vasculitis. This could be anything, even just ordinary dysentery or food poisoning. I phoned Ross with the negative news.

'She's much worse today. Vomiting now and her albumen is dropping. I think she's now got involvement of the duodenum and small bowel. I'm just going to pop the scope down from the other side and have a look at her upper gut and small bowel. I'll get some duodenal biopsies for you to look at.'

I looked at Achara's blood results. They were terrible and, as Ross said, they were getting worse.

'What's that?' Alex the senior registrar had brought Achara's slides to re-examine on the double-headed microscope with me. 'Down in the corner of that last level? I've marked it.' Alex sure had very sharp eyes. I had missed it, for there, burrowed deeply into the bowel wall, was a creature. When I cut deeper levels in, it became quite a big creature, too. Not a bacterium, but a parasite of some sort.

'What on earth is it? I just don't recognise it.'

I had seen many parasites in Africa, but never one mining down this deep into the bowel. We leafed through the books on tropical parasites, but I just couldn't quite get it to fit any of the pictures. The best fit was a female pin worm, but why?

These were usually harmless and only caused an annoying anal itching — hardly that serious, and certainly not in the league of what was happening to this patient.

'She has got a very high level of eosinophils in her blood. Nearly 20 per cent. I'd put that down to the vasculitis. But maybe she's got some rare, invasive parasite?'

The answer came with the duodenal biopsies.

'Look!'

We all saw it at once and exclaimed together. There, living in the crypts of the bowel, were numerous adult worms. We could see their muscular, larval offspring swarming off the surface, while their aggressive needle-shaped young punched their bore holes deeply into the bowel wall. Achara's body was fighting back with its white cells, but the worms were clearly and overwhelmingly winning this battle. Now at last we could recognise the culprits.

'It's strongyloides!' I said, for they were now easy to recognise. 'It's a hyper-infection because of her low-immunity status.'

Bruce Lockett nodded his head in agreement.

'What's happened?' The young registrars were alongside us, looking at what we were looking at.

'It's strongyloides, a round worm that normally lives quietly in the bowel and doesn't cause too many serious problems. The body sort of keeps it corralled in there. Achara has certainly picked up this infestation in Thailand and now it's gone wild, as she's on immunosuppressive drugs. Her immune system just can't hold them at bay. The worms are colonising the gut, laying eggs, and their hatchling larvae are massively invading the bowel. Achara's blood has got nothing to fight back with!'

'Listen to this!' Alex was reading *Pathology of Tropical and Extraordinary Diseases*. 'It's disgusting! The larvae are usually in the soil and get into the blood by penetrating the skin. They go to the lungs where the worms develop. Then you cough them up and swallow them down alive! That's how they get to the bowel! I think I feel sick!'

'Better phone Ross with the news now. The patient needs to stop her immunosuppressive drugs and get started on anti-parasitic treatment urgently.'

Sadly, even as we were making the diagnosis, Achara died of septicaemia and shock. We just hadn't picked this up fast enough. A pathologist's discovery of the correct diagnosis in life is only really helpful when we find a treatable disease, but we also have to do it in time for the treatment to work. Too often, as in Achara's case, I have run as fast as I could to catch a patient's diagnostic bus, only to see the doors slam shut and to be left on the pavement, ruefully watching it drive off to another place. A place from which no-one returns. It's an old joke that pathologists know all the answers, only too late.

Alas, that is sometimes the way of it in medicine.

Achara Nok. 13 May 2014. Requiescat in pace.

* * *

Sometimes, though, we do get it very right and we're able to make a difference.

'I have a problem I'd like to talk to you about.'

Bill is a Whanganui-based GP, with a perceptive and inquiring mind. He's often on the phone discussing his patients' results and challenging us to come up with a diagnosis. This time it was a little different.

'Sure, Bill. What's the story?'

'I have a personal problem that I need help with. I've got diarrhoea. It's appalling and I've had it since 1990. I have some days when I have up to six explosive, watery motions with vast amounts of wind. When it comes it's urgent and I've got to get to a toilet damn fast. Some days aren't so bad. But it always comes back. Lately, it seems it's getting worse and I'm also getting nausea and painful colic, too.'

He paused.

'It's a real challenge to drive from Whanganui to Palmerston North. It's only 50 minutes, but I have to plan stops along the way in Turakina and Bulls and Sanson. I know every public lavatory in the lower North Island pretty well by now, I can tell you.'

'God, that's dreadful! Twelve years! Sounds pretty devastating. Have you cultured for bacteria and sent stools for us to look for parasites?'

'Oh, yes. Many times. Everything is negative. I also saw a professor in Wellington and he did an endoscopy and biopsied my stomach and duodenum.'

'What did they find? I'm guessing it wasn't coeliac disease in the duodenum, otherwise you wouldn't be here asking me.'

'Both biopsies were reported as normal and my coeliac antibodies are negative. That was four years ago. Can you get my slides and review them to see if there's anything there? I'm really desperate and it's interfering with my practice. Sometimes I have to leave the surgery in the middle of seeing a patient and rush home. It's so bad I'm seriously thinking of retiring three years early, but I really don't want to. I'm going to get a second opinion from specialists in Auckland, too.'

'Of course I will. What year did you have the biopsies?'

'The biopsies were in 1998.'

The package containing Bill's slides arrived later in the week. There were plenty of them. Biopsies had been taken from the stomach, the duodenum, the terminal ileum and all along the colon and rectum. I studied them carefully and they all looked more or less normal. Except for the duodenum where something caught my eye.

Normally, the cells lining the duodenum stand immaculately arrayed side by side, just like a line of Grenadier Guards. Bill's lining was just too cellular and didn't look quite right. It was here that I saw small, dark lymphocytes infiltrating the lining between the cells. It was as if that imaginary line of rigid Grenadier Guards had been overrun by a clambering troop of hundreds of monkeys. I carried out a test and marked the invading cells. They were all T-lymphocytes, the inflammatory cells of the body. They shouldn't have been there. What were they up to? Answer that question, I thought, and we'd know what Bill's problem was.

'What can cause this?' Bill asked, when I phoned him for more information. 'Do you know?'

He sounded desperate to me.

'Lots of things can. We just have to work through them. It's found in patients with coeliac disease who are on a strict, gluten-free diet. Their lining becomes normal but the lymphocytes stay behind. You sometimes also get it in the families of coeliacs.'

'No. I'm not on a gluten-free diet and I haven't got any family history of coeliac disease.'

'What about other food allergies? Lymphocytosis has also been found in people with allergies to milk, eggs and tuna fish.'

'I've hardly ever had tuna. I had an appalling attack all through one night after eating a meal of mussels, but I avoid shellfish like the plague now, of course. I could try avoiding eggs and milk, I suppose.'

'And there's tropical sprue. But that doesn't apply here in New Zealand, as you have to be within 38 degrees of the equator.'

There was a short pause on the other end of the phone.

'Didn't I tell you the diarrhoea started in the Philippines?'

'No! I wasn't aware of that. Now *that* is interesting.'

'I was a missionary in Manila for eight years, you know. I had a cast-iron gut before I went there. That's where it all started and it's never stopped since.'

'Where did you get your water from?'

'A pretty terrible well. The water wasn't treated in any way. Could that be the source?'

'It's certainly possible. No-one has found the organism or organisms that cause tropical sprue. Whatever it is, it's an elusive creature. But it's there, all right. Doxycycline cures it, but it may take a bit of time to knock it out.'

It was a little while before I heard from Bill again. One day he dropped in to see me.

'While I was waiting to go for my Auckland appointment, I stopped eggs and then dairy foods for a couple of weeks and then reintroduced them to my diet again. No significant benefit. So food allergy didn't seem likely.'

Bill shook his head ruefully. I wasn't surprised. I'd never come across a food allergy with quite the serious effects he was showing.

'Six days before going to Auckland I decided to treat for tropical sprue and I began doxycycline. Within two days I felt great and my motions were 90 per cent normal. After four weeks, this continues to be the case, for which I am immensely grateful. Retirement is not now on the short-term agenda as it was a couple of months ago. I suppose the lesson is to get second opinions on histology if there's any doubt about the diagnosis.'

Bill went happily on his way. I was touched to receive a hamper of fine wines, cheeses and biscuits by way of thanks. It's rare for pathologists ever to be appreciated by our patients, even the live ones — we're the specialists' specialists, and we're largely invisible to those whose cases we consider.

When I was a fourth-year medical student in Rhodesia, I was a guinea pig in an investigation designed to find tropical sprue's culprit bug. I was one of the 'normal' subjects: I had to swallow a substantial piece of hardware called a Crosby capsule, which was attached to a long, large-calibre, clear, plastic tube, and let it sit in my gut for three hours. Those three hours were horribly uncomfortable. I retched throughout, my body trying to vomit the thick, hard pipe from my gullet. My eyes watered with the effort and I felt dreadful. It certainly wasn't worth the $15 I was paid! From time to time, the people performing the procedure checked via X-ray to see whether my stomach had passed the capsule into my duodenum. As soon as it had, they sucked bowel lining into the capsule and triggered a little guillotine that lopped off a bit of my bowel lining. The whole apparatus was then retracted, complete with my bit of bowel, which was then sent off for analysis.

I thought *I'd* had it badly. The Crosby capsule fell off its tether when it was being withdrawn from the student who came after me. He was sent home with instructions to collect his stools over the following days and sieve them until he found the capsule: it was an expensive item, you see, and nothing was disposable in those days.

So what did they find from my and others' ghastly experience? Nothing at all. No bugs were identifiable in either patients with tropical sprue or in us normal medical student controls. That was hardly surprising back then. But it seems strange in the age of flexible endoscopes (which give easy access to the gut from above and below without the need for Crosby capsules) and sophisticated labs, with the ability to culture just about anything and to perform DNA probes, that the offending bug is still elusive. Fortunately, it doesn't matter so much, because tetracycline antibiotics kill it outright.

And herein lies the terrible tragedy of this story. Bill's 12 years of debilitating diarrhoea could have been avoided with a short course of cheap antibiotics. Imagine spending 12 long years of your life with the unrelenting runs: it's just too horrible to contemplate.

* * *

'I've got a problem specimen here.'

I was in my office. Talia was calling from the cut-up room, where the registrars daily dissected the organs and biopsy specimens sent from the theatres, the procedure rooms, the clinics and GPs' surgeries. There were thirty-five thousand of them every year, and anything could pitch up.

'What's up?' I asked. Talia was pretty experienced. This would be something genuinely odd.

'It's a parasite that a GP has removed from a man's scalp. He's been travelling around Vietnam, Thailand and Laos.'

'That's weird. Is it a round, maggoty thing?' Even as I asked, I shuddered, thinking of putzi fly warbles.

'Not really. It's all broken up, greyish-white and shiny. I just don't recognise it as a parasite at all.'

I was intrigued. I went to investigate.

We stood, puzzled, around the bench staring down at the fragmented specimen. It looked like nothing on earth that I had ever seen.

'It's a bit slimy.' I touched it gingerly with my bare finger and pulled away hastily. I looked guiltily around. This was setting a bad example. I knew I was supposed to wear gloves. God only knows how infectious or toxic any of our unknown specimens were. 'I really haven't a clue what it is. All I know is that it's bigger than a 50-cent piece and I don't know of any parasite that size that can burrow into the skin. Process it and let's have a look under the microscope. Maybe then we'll know.'

It was beautiful to behold the stained slide. As I focused on it the next morning, a wonderful world of microscopic chaos came into view. It was like a particularly lovely kaleidoscope. It wouldn't have been out of place in the MONA or the Tate Modern galleries. There were sheets of thick-walled, irregularly patterned lattices; tubules holding minute, pigmented plates in long, even stacks; irregular vessels coursing through; and hollowed, densely coated spherules stuffed full of light-orange granules.

'Is it a putzi fly maggot?'

I shook my head. I was puzzled. 'Definitely not. I'm not even sure if it's an animal. It looks like an alien.' I smiled, and lowered my voice. "'It is not life as we know or understand it. Yet it is obviously alive. It exists.'"

The registrars looked back at me blankly.

'Spock?' I said. 'Fom the original *Star Trek*? Surely you've heard that saying before?'

More blank looks.

'You've heard of *Star Trek*, haven't you?'

'Of course we have!' they shot back at me. 'But no-one watches that ancient first series any more.'

I sighed and shook my head. The younger generation. What did they know? I just despaired.

'There are a few fragments of human skin here, but they look as if they've been scratched off the surface. There's no inflammation or blood in here. Are you sure the GP removed this from the scalp? It's an enormous creature for a start and there's just no inflammatory reaction to it. Not an attacking white cell anywhere to say the body is going after it, is there?'

'That's what the request form says: "Parasite removed from scalp. Has travelled to Vietnam, Thailand and Laos." Seems quite clear.' Talia held the paper up for us to see.

I just had to phone the GP and find out. The GP was surprised.

'No, I don't know anything about this. I didn't even know there were any specimens. I certainly didn't cut it out. The patient developed intense itching after their trip and was absolutely certain there were worms emerging from his scalp. His wife confirms it all. She says she's seen them herself. I couldn't see anything there except scratch marks. I just gave them the form and a pot to collect them in. They were supposed to bring them in here for me to examine, not take them to the lab.'

'Have they ever brought in any of these worms for you to see?' I was intrigued. It seemed unlikely, but stranger things have happened.

'Oh yes, several times. They just looked like bits of bark and apple and hair to me so I didn't send them in. I've treated him with permethrin for scabies and I'm wondering whether to prescribe an antihelminthic for worms? And I've booked him in to see the dermatologist.'

'No. I wouldn't give any medications at this stage. Let us see what we can make of this first.'

Bruce Lockett came in and registered the tight knot of medical professionals around the examination bench at once.

'What are you all looking at?'

We told him the story. He took one look at it and knew what it was.

'This is a plant, or blended-up bits of a plant. It's got a strange anatomy, but it's phloem and xylem or bits of stamens or something. But those rigid walls are quite unmistakable. Do a PAS stain and you'll see the cellulose will stain up purple.'

The periodic acid–Schiff or PAS stain is a test we routinely use to detect polysaccharides, of which the cellulose of plant walls is but one.

'A plant?' mused Stephen, one of the pathology registrars. 'He must be in the police force then.'

It was my turn to look blank.

'A member of Special Branch?' he murmured.

Sometimes even weak humour is funny. We all laughed. Something clicked in my mind.

'I remember a similar case about ten years ago. He was a patient in the medical ward and he was convinced he had parasites in his hair. He was often in here combing out his hair onto sheets of white paper. There was never anything there but debris and dandruff. His doctor said it was Morgellons disease, I think. I can't remember the patient's name but I think he eventually responded to treatment. Anyway, he stopped bringing us in the bits and pieces of rubbish.'

No sooner had I dropped the name 'Morgellons disease' than the registrars were busy on their phones.

'Morgellons disease. Worms of the brain, it says here. Dr Google says it's also called delusional parasitosis. The patients seek non-psychiatric medical help and if the infestation is denied they can become hostile or even violent.'

'I think that's what this must be. It sounds a horrible problem. I know how bad I felt when I had the putzi maggots, and that was disgusting enough. It must be even worse for this poor man, I reckon. Real or imaginary, it doesn't make any difference. I'd better let the GP know. There's little point wasting a dermatologist's time and the sooner they get the psychiatrists onto treating this poor soul the better.'

CHAPTER 4

Earth to Earth, Ashes to Ashes, Dust to Dust

Flies are a curse. We may not have horrors like putzi flies laying their eggs in our living flesh in New Zealand, but we do have blowflies. I'm sure you're well acquainted with them. They arrive in the summertime, tagging along in ones and twos with the more numerous droves of newly hatched house flies that swarm into our houses. House flies are bad enough. I have a private theory that they're summoned by the aroma of the neighbourhood barbecues. They buzz in circles in the middle of a room and alight on every table, on every plate, on every scrap of food where they spot their crap on each and every surface. They won't go away. They drive me mad — mad enough to start a wholesale slaughter with the swatter. But no amount of execution seems to dent their numbers at all. And the swatter itself seems no match for blowflies, which take blows that would deal death to a dozen of their lesser companions. I have a particular loathing for them, and I meet them professionally, too, all the time.

Blowflies are also aptly known as carrion flies. The smell of death is the aroma of the elixir of life to them, because their life cycle depends upon their finding dead flesh. Like the African vulture, blowflies have an exquisitely sensitive ability to see, smell or perhaps even to divine the presence of death. They come so quickly that I wonder that the departure of the soul releases some dark pheromone drawing them to the waiting feast. The soft, moist tissue of lifeless eyes of any exposed corpse will soon be decorated with bandoliers of white flecks like tiny grains of rice. Hours later, the eggs will have hatched into hordes of writhing maggots which fan out to find their way into the body's cavities.

They have often been companions in my work, particularly when a body is discovered in a state of advanced decay. Decayed bodies pop up more commonly than they should in a country such as New Zealand. It's understandable when the bodies are the victims of poorly concealed murders or of accidents in remote places. It is much harder to accept when they're found within the homes of our populous cities and towns.

I had just finished my morning coffee. I had picked up the materials relating to a case of gastric cancer that I wanted to show and discuss with the surgeons at our lunchtime clinico-pathological conference, when the phone rang. It was the police. A detective sergeant identified himself.

'Gidday. Sorry to trouble you, Doc, but we've located a body we'd like you to have a look at.'

I looked at my watch. The surgical meeting had just gone out the window.

'Where is it?' Please let it not be way out in the bush, or hours of toil up in the mountains.

'In a room at the Cedar Lodge.'

I knew the place. Cedar Lodge was only a few blocks from the hospital. It was sometimes unkindly known as the Seedy Lodge — a small, low-budget residential hotel, with a clientele of pensioners, itinerants and the usual town and city dwellers who found themselves with nowhere else to stay.

'What's happened? Does it look suspicious?'

'Nah, not really. Been dead a little while, I reckon. Just want you to have a look and see if there's anything to worry about.'

'I'll be there in ten minutes.'

I nodded to myself. This was going to be nothing, I was sure. Who knows? Perhaps I could even be back in time for the surgical meeting.

I turned into North Street and pulled up opposite the Cedar Lodge. You can always get parking close by your destination around Palmerston North. I started to open my door and stopped.

And stared.

There, sitting on my windscreen, was the biggest blowfly I have ever seen. It was iridescent in the sunlight and its hairs waved like a stiff quiff in the breeze. I knew instinctively that he was the outrider of a bigger clan gathered close by. I knew he had everything to do with why I was there.

I climbed out, pulling my investigation bag behind me. The smell hit me immediately, even though I was parked a little way down the street. It wasn't overwhelming but it was there, catarrhal and thick enough to be hardly distinguishable from a taste. I grimaced. This was not going to be easy.

The detective sergeant was waiting at the door. He seemed unperturbed by the odour.

'He's up here, Doc. We know who he is but haven't got a confirmed visual identification yet. He's just lying on the bed in his clothes.'

'Any past record?'

Perhaps he was a known drug dealer, although it seemed far more likely he would be a drug user. Only a very unsuccessful dealer would live in the Cedar Lodge.

'Nah. Unemployed on a sickness benefit. Hangs around town but no criminal history with us. Goes to some clinic up in the hospital.'

'Likely a medical cause of death, then. I'll check his notes when I get back to the hospital.'

I followed the policeman in. The air was even thicker and fouler here. I felt a wave of nausea starting in my midriff and quickly suppressed it. We went into the hotel foyer. Off to one side was the dining room with about a dozen tables set for lunch. I stopped and looked in disbelief. Every table was full. The guests were eating their lunch and with some relish, I thought. Could they not smell that awful and quite unmistakable odour of a decaying human being?

I followed slowly, my heart heavy, up the stairs to the first level. A uniformed constable stood guard in the passageway. He looked pretty uneasy to me. It was a warm day to be sure, but he had a patina of sickly dampness about his face and neck. Here, I thought, giving him a sympathetic nod, is someone else who can smell this miasma of death hovering over us.

I took a deep breath and entered a simple but untidy room. There was an unmade bed against the wall, on which lay a bundle of old washing. At my appearance, a cloud of blowflies rose from the washing and angrily circled, buzzing their displeasure. The bundle of washing slowly resolved into the corpse of a fully clothed man, partly covered by blankets and with his face to the wall.

I peeled the blanket back, wincing as the trapped gases were released. The urge to vomit was back, and stronger than before: I gritted my teeth as saliva flooded my mouth. I climbed onto the bed and with difficulty leaned over the corpse to perform my examination. I steadied myself on the windowsill as I peered down into his face and then studied his body. His pants were hitched up and crumpled. A pair of pilled, crusted socks covered his feet. His skin was marbled grey and blue.

My unveiling of the body had re-energised the flies buzzing at the window. Several blowflies, recognisable as the kith and kin of the scout squatting on my car windscreen, took turns buzzing and bumping at the warmth of the windowpane. They had done their duty and laid their eggs and now they only wanted out.

His face was a dirty cream colour, unshaven, unwashed and marked with signs of poor health. The jaw hung slackly, the upper crusty dental plate dropped down like a portcullis. His breath may long since have been stilled by death but it still was foetid down there. I easily pushed the jaw closed to cover the horror of the mouth. So there was no rigor mortis here: more than 72 hours since death, I thought automatically, although his state of decay did make that kind of obvious.

'There's nothing suspicious here that I can see,' I said, climbing off the bed, straightening and turning away. 'There are no visible injuries and he's not been tied up or anything like that. Best get him to the mortuary so these people,'

I nodded towards the door in the direction of the rest of the hotel guests, 'can have their meals without that bloody awful stink. How the hell can they just sit there and put up with it?'

'I've seen it before,' said the detective, shrugging. 'It's funny how you can get used to a smell. It happens all the time with bodies stuck in flats in the city and the neighbours just don't even notice.'

'I suppose if it starts gradually enough you could get used to it,' I agreed. 'I've read that in the trenches in the First World War they lived with the smell permanently. The soldiers got so used to it that they could eat happily enough despite decayed body parts being thrown up all around them by shellfire.'

We went downstairs. The air did seem rather easier here, despite the disturbance that my investigations must have caused. I noticed the guests had now started on their pudding.

Back in the mortuary, we can deal with decayed bodies much more easily than in a public hotel. A laminar flow changes the whole roomful of air six times a minute, and we've got pretty good masks and scrubs and waterproof gear to cover up. Though, of course, it isn't just water that we have to worry about proofing ourselves against, is it? It's blood and body juices, rancid liquid fat, faeces and fluids mostly, and, believe me, it all leaks and seeps into every crevice.

Larry Hall was several days into his decomposition cycle when we got him stripped and on the gurney. His stomach wall was like a picture with a frame of verdant green. In life, the flora of his bowel were quiet and model citizens. Now, they had emerged for a final feast on the cadaver and their sulphide wastes stained the skin along the course of the deeper colon.

His veins were beautifully etched on his grubby skin, charcoal on cream, a delicate lattice of marble. Indeed, we call this effect 'marbling', and it marks the steady tramp of bacterial putrefaction through the veins from the bowel across the surface of the skin. When I touched his flank, the skin slid smoothly off the body as a sheet, exposing weeping, pink, raw and discoloured flesh. This slippage has a slimy and disgusting feel and it occurs when the anchors of the skin finally liquefy and it loses its grip on the body it has so faithfully protected in life. Rafts of blowfly eggs were there, too, of course, decorating the corners of the eyes, just about where you rub the crusted sleep from your half-closed eyes when you wake each morning.

Thankfully, no maggots had yet hatched. I hate working amongst those crawling little bastards.

The signs indicated he had died six to seven days before. Weird 'body farms' have been established in the United States precisely so that the timing of the changes of decay can be studied. Even so, the exact timing depends on a range of factors. Larry was indoors and warm, covered in blankets, so the onset of putrefaction was a lot faster than it would have been outside in the winter. So that was about the best I could do for the time of death.

I had to work hard to find the cause of death. Larry was well known to the hospital, where he was periodically seen in the respiratory clinic with pretty advanced obstructive airway disease causing bad scarring of his lungs. I could see Ken, the mortuary assistant, struggling and getting more and more frustrated at the lungs, which began to rip apart as he pulled at them. Old pleurisy had gummed them hard and tight to the ribs, the heart, the spine and the breastbone. Ken was quite volatile and tended to rush in flailing and ripping when things weren't going right.

'Stop!' I said. I couldn't watch this kind of damage to a body, no matter how scarred. 'Here. Let me do it!'

He was reluctant, but I pushed him aside and started dissecting the fibrous scar with a scalpel a few millimetres at a time. It was a tiring and demanding task, like working inside a deep barrel as I made my way into the chest cavity slowly freeing up the lungs. An hour passed and my mask was becoming horribly uncomfortable as its fibres tickled my nose. I couldn't bear it and without thinking I reached up and rubbed my nose.

Big mistake.

My mask was a cloth one and it was hot and wet with my breath and my rubber glove was glistening with fats and foul body fluids. Their thick odour, more like a taste, flooded through the damp fabric of the mask instantly.

I leapt back and ripped the mask from my face in disgust.

Second mistake.

I should have taken my glove off first, shouldn't I? For all I did was now smear the same ordure over my face where I had grabbed the mask. Ken laughed at my discomfort. I reckon he was glad I had taken over the terrible task.

After a wash and a change of gear, I went back to work and eventually pulled the chest organs out and laid them on the dissection table. The lungs were slimy with decomposition and surprisingly hard to get a good grip on while I sliced them open with my long dissection knife. I sliced along the length of the left lung and felt the firm scar tissue beneath, the sign of a host of old infections. The organ flapped open and there was the answer. A log of blood clot the colour of dark chocolate was blocking a large branch of the left pulmonary artery. A pulmonary embolism. This often causes instant death, as the block prevents blood reaching the lungs and then stops the heart filling, so that the whole pump and bellows of life are disconnected.

The clot must have come from his pelvis or maybe from his legs, but I couldn't find the origin. It was late, my new mask was also beginning to itch and a long and difficult dissection deep in the bowl of a pelvis awash with rank fluid held little appeal. Maybe it had started originally there in life and entirely broke away in the rush of the bloodstream, or maybe it had come from somewhere else. It didn't really matter where it came from: all that mattered was where it ended up, blocking the lung, which is what killed Larry Hall.

There is always sorrow in death, even for those of us who are in its presence every day of our working lives. For the likes of Larry Hall, I also feel a sort of 'if only' kind of sorrow: if only he had done something a little differently long ago, maybe he wouldn't have died unmourned, unloved and unmissed. We once kept a man's body in our mortuary fridge for three months. He'd died in hospital where his death certificate was signed by a house surgeon, so the coroner had no legal interest in him. We waited and waited for the funeral directors to come and take him for burial or cremation, as always happens.

No-one came. No-one seemed to know. No-one seemed to care.

No-one did anything until Pat, the mortuary head technician, one day said: 'He's been here a long time. When are they going to pick him up?'

We found out he had no family at all and no friends. He lived alone in a run-down house in Levin. The police were sent to the house, where they found the lights on and the radio playing, as it had continuously for the past three months. No-one had heard, checked or cared. God alone knows what his letterbox must have looked like. His pension kept being paid and his rent was deducted automatically. He might have stayed in our fridge for years if Pat hadn't said anything — although it would have to have been decades to break any sort of record.

We're horrified when we hear of bodies lying unseen amongst us for weeks and months, and each time we hear of such a story, there's a collective belief that we should somehow do better. Care more. Get to know your neighbours and check on them, we're told.

But we don't, do we? You don't have to be old or a recluse to go missing but not be missed. It seems quite unbelievable that a 19-year-old student of Canterbury University lay dead and undiscovered for four weeks in the Sonoda hall of residence in Christchurch. When he was eventually found in September 2019, the university authorities said it was 'inconceivable'. But it was not only conceivable: it happened, and it will happen again.

In 1966, a Croatian woman, Hedviga Golik, sat down with a cup of tea to watch a television programme on her valve-driven, black-and-white TV set. Some time before the end of the show, she died. She had sat there, dead and undisturbed, way past the end of the show, through vast global changes and even as rockets and cluster bombs rained down upon her neighbourhood. It was 2008 — fully 42 years — before her body was found, still sitting there, lightly shrouded with

The Quick and the Dead

cobwebs. In all that time, no-one had called or checked up on her, although her relatives had reported her missing way back in 1966.

When I heard that story, I wondered how long it was before the television valves finally flickered and they, too, died?

Larry Hall. August 1992. Requiescat in pace.

* * *

Christmas 2001 was coming. All the excitement around the millennium had long since abated: the clock had ticked over midnight, 2000, and the world still spun on its axis, the sun rose punctually in the east just as it had for millions of years already. I was struggling with the annual problem all husbands have. What on earth could I buy Elayne for Christmas? I had no idea where to begin looking and there was only two weeks to go. The pressure gnawed at me. And today, the 11th of December, was our wedding anniversary. We were going out for a celebratory dinner.

The phone rang. I snatched it up. It was Jeanette Parks.

Jeanette is a wonderful detective with whom we worked closely. She's small of stature, has masses of thick, curly, red hair and a smile that could launch ships. Amongst her many accomplishments, she's a highly skilled hunter on horseback. We all loved Jeanette and her bright mind and quick wit.

'What's up, Jeanette?' She never messed us around, so I knew a call from her was important.

'Got a decomp for you out beyond Halcombe.'

'Oh.'

A decomp was a decomposed corpse.

All of a sudden, my mouth was full of saliva and a foul taste — completely psychosomatic, but there all the same. I swallowed the disgust, but my mood dimmed several shades. Where the hell was Halcombe, anyway? I had an idea it was way out beyond Feilding. Bugger.

'Yep. Don't think we've got a murder here, but you do need to see this.'

I loaded up my pathology registrars, Stephen and Kate, and we set off for the rural back-blocks of the Manawatu. After the usual aimless and irritating meander amongst the identical, unmarked rural-type proto-roads, we found Tokorangi Road and there, by the roadside, our destination became immediately obvious.

A solitary police car stood sentinel on the road. It blocked half the carriageway as the roadside ditches were so steep that you dared not pull in too close to the verge. Not that it mattered: there was minimal traffic. We pulled up behind the police car.

Murder scenes are a bustle of activity, by contrast with this one. There was only the one car and Jeanette waiting at the gate. She laughed at the sight of us. I fleetingly wondered why, but decided it must have been because we all enjoyed each other's company so much.

'So, what surprises do you have tucked away for us?' I asked. We stood by the gate as Jeanette pulled her notebook from behind her stab-proof vest. Even back then the police were wearing them routinely.

'Ed Laurence is a retired, divorced farmer living on his own. He's been down at the hospital in Palmy for all sorts of problems. God knows what they are.' Jeanette flashed her brilliant smile at us. 'Anyway, no-one checks up on him regularly, apparently. Lots of mail in his box.' Jeanette pointed at the crammed letterbox. 'Copies of the *Guardian* going back a month plus other crap. Rural area here, so no-one would even notice.'

'So he's probably about a month gone? Is it really bad in there?' My mind was already messing with my body and the very thought of what might be waiting made me feel like vomiting on the spot.

But Jeanette's face was untroubled. She smiled knowingly at us.

'Just go up and have a look. He's in the bedroom. Duncan has set up stepping plates for you.'

Detective Duncan Taylor was Jeanette's partner in the force. Duncan was a tall cop, one of the tallest, as I remember him. He had a great sense of humour, but he was deadly serious about his work, a true professional, the best type of provincial policeman. The perfect foil for Jeanette, really. They were the long and the short of it.

We went in with some trepidation. I was in my usual jacket and tie, as befitted my status as a consultant. Kate was in a summer dress with sandals, Stephen with his Doc Martens boots but otherwise unmemorably attired, as we boys often tend to be.

I was sure now that Jeanette was laughing at us about something. I felt suspicious and uneasy.

Duncan had placed the first stepping plate just inside the front door. The second was a good metre beyond that and the third equally further on. These may have been small steps for Duncan's great stride but they were great leaps for me and I am six foot tall.

I leapt to the next plate and landed with a crash. Kate and Stephen followed behind. They are both shorter than me but were managing as nimbly as a pair of high-school triple jumpers. We followed the trail of plates into the passage. We were still five metres from the bedroom door when I looked down.

It was ghastly. The carpet was heaving with maggots. Fat bloated maggots. Their segmented bodies pulsed, stretching out until they were half their usual diameter, latching onto the carpet fibres at their front and then telescoping their bodies forward. They had already travelled a vast distance from where they had been born, metres away down the hall, with this pulsatile motion. Relative to their size, it would be about the same as you and me walking the 70 kilometres from Palmerston North to Whanganui.

Disgustingly, they were already hauling their eager, maggoty bodies up the sides and over the tops of the stepping plates. I had crushed several beneath my shoes, their smeared entrails contaminating the anti-slip ribbing of the plates. I felt sick at the thought of those burst maggots I was mushing beneath the soles of my shoes.

There was nothing to be done but continue jumping from one plate to the next, ignoring the grubs underfoot. Duncan was there waiting for us in the bedroom.

'Gidday, Doc.' He nodded at Stephen and Kate. They, too, were well known by now to the Manawatu police. 'There he is.' Duncan pointed at the bed.

I looked curiously. There was surprisingly little smell. The drifting, dense miasma of putrefaction had largely gone, replaced by an almost savoury aroma. A skull covered by dry, yellowish, parchment-like skin lay on the pillow, the sockets staring sightlessly at the ceiling. The bedclothes were drawn up covering the body, but the arms lay on top at rest. The man had clearly been in a state of repose when he died. I moved closer. There was a large and impressive watch on the left wrist, but I noticed it had stopped at twenty to three. There was a necklace pendant around the neck.

'Looks pretty natural, doesn't it?' I said, turning to Duncan. He nodded.

'The house is secure and there's no sign of a forced entry,' he told us. 'There doesn't seem to be anything obviously missing or disturbed. He was found by a friend from Halcombe who dropped in to check on him. He's been in poor health for a while, apparently.'

Kate shrieked and swore. We looked at her in astonishment. She was vigorously shaking her feet.

'The little bastards are climbing me!' We looked down at her feet and so they were. The maggots were avidly scaling the sides of her open sandals and wriggling over her feet. I looked at mine. They were there, too, but closed shoes and socks didn't seem to appeal to them as much as bare flesh. I suppose they were starving, looking for a fresh source of food, for they had sure as hell completely cleaned up the man lying there in the bed.

Maggots will eat the living, too, of course. In rural New Zealand they lay their eggs around a sheep's arse, where they will harvest the merest specks of shit on which to feast and grow. And they will voraciously attack the slightest skin scratch and then devour it away to make a huge rotting hole. They will do the same to people, colonising the neglected elderly or infants in the same way. They have the tools for the job too. They poo a toxic brew of enzymes over any wound to break down the flesh, which they then grind to mince with rows of hard, sharp hooks lining their mouths. They are the least gracious of diners, eating off the very table on which they have also crapped.

I shook the bastards off my feet but fresh waves began their assault. Belatedly, I realised why Jeanette was laughing at us when we arrived. She knew exactly what would happen to us inside. I had better make this as quick as possible so we could get clear of these dreadful creatures.

I moved to the side of the bed. Here the bedding and the floor were darkly stained where the purging of his body fluids had occurred, gushing out as the corpse swelled with the gases of decay. I pulled back the bedding. Surprisingly little smell wafted from beneath the covers.

The whole body was skeletonised. A fresh tide of maggots disturbed by the sudden light swept out from inside the body and spilled out over the covers, adding to the thousands and thousands in the room. He was still wearing his pyjamas.

'Collect some of the maggots into a couple of containers,' I said to Stephen. 'Maybe we can get them dated and get a rough time of death. The experts apparently can figure out what stage they're at and calculate the number of days since hatching, giving a rough post-mortem interval.'

'Can you do us a Life Extinct certificate?' Jeanette asked us, still grinning, when we got outside. We could. There was no doubt that life was extinct. But what was the cause of death?

The autopsy was unrevealing, with only 24 kilograms of bone left behind by the feeding flies. There were no bone fractures to suggest an assault. The lumbar spine was twisted into an S-shape but that was just an old malformation he'd had all his life.

It is often the case with skeletal remains that there is little to find on which to re-create the story of the final passage into death. This case became memorable for the wrong reason. It was either Jeanette or Kate who suggested we wind up Duncan. It was part of our 'black humour'.

'Tell him it's not a natural death. Tell him it's a murder,' I was asked.

He had already arranged for the house to be decontaminated and disinfected. If this were a murder there would be hell to pay with any evidence now obliterated. Being of a naturally mischievous disposition, I went along with it. I called Duncan.

'Bad news, mate,' I said to him. 'This could be a homicide.'

'Why? What's happened?' Duncan's voice was at once high and tense. He was worried, I could tell. I knew the industrial cleaners were even then at work on the house.

'Fractured skull, mate. Doesn't look good. You didn't drop him bringing him out, did you?'

He was really anxious. I strung him along for a bit, but eventually I took pity on him and told him all was okay. It was a natural cause of death.

We all laughed at this. It wasn't at all disrespectful to my deceased patient, Ed. I guess in this job we need to find humour and levity where we can. Otherwise the shocking sights you see will just get you down in the end. Humour — one of humanity's defining qualities — is the best antidote. I reckon we need a lot more of it.

But the punchline to this story was as unfunny as it gets. Duncan came into the mortuary soon after this episode, but under very different circumstances. That is another story.

We finally figured out Ed's cause of death by consulting

his history. He'd had surgery on his right foot to release a trapped nerve and as a result of this he had developed a clot in the veins of his leg. These deep vein thromboses after surgery are a real nuisance and can be fatal. Ed was put on warfarin to dampen down the clotting factors in his blood. When it works, this treatment stops the clot spreading to other veins and, much more importantly, stops the growth of a tail of fresh thrombus hanging freely off the back of the clot. This tail can break off and travel to the lungs to cause a fatal embolism, just as had happened to Larry Hall. The blood thinners never give 100 per cent protection, and odds are that it must have been a pulmonary embolism that killed him as he lay there in his bed. That was my best guess, as I explained to the coroner. It had to be a guess, because the ultimate evidence of the clot had disappeared out the window on the wings of the carrion flies.

Even with the organs all still there, the story sometimes — often, even — still remains a mystery with decomposed bodies. In such circumstances, 'obscure natural causes' is the unsatisfactory best that we can offer to the coroner and to the family.

Ed Laurence. November 2001. Requiescat in pace.

CHAPTER 5

The Meat-Eaters

'Mail for you.' The department secretary handed me an envelope. It had a stamp and my name and address were handwritten on it. These days, that sort of letter is a real rarity, so my interest was piqued. I turned it over. There was the return address. Very old-fashioned but impressive and very properly executed, much as I had been taught to do when I was at school last century.

It was from Dr Nick Thomson, I saw. I knew of Nick when he was a well-known and highly respected GP in Hunterville, though he had retired some years before. We had recently met at a talk where he had told me the story of a strange case with which he had been closely involved. I was intrigued by his tale and asked him for the details: here they were and, as a treat, they were arriving by old-fashioned snail-mail. I slit the envelope and read the contents with interest.

'I was a mission doctor at Iruna in Papua New Guinea for eight years. There were six of us overseas staff on the mission and the minister was David Clarke, who was an Australian. It was a vast territory to cover with so few of us on the ground but we did our best. David decided it was time to minister to the western end of our district and he flew out to Robinson River to visit the far-flung congregations and converts there.

'David had given us the date when he would be back and we were not concerned at all for him. This was, after all, a routine trip. But he didn't come back on the day he had told us, or even on the next. Then I became worried and started to look for him, even though travel delays are not uncommon out there.'

I could understand this. In the wilder parts of the globe, travel is often complicated and things often don't run on the precise timing we've come to expect in the developed world.

'The evidence I collected of his journey is fragmentary and I have put together as best I can the stories from the local pastors along his route.

'David had a long and hard haul along the coastal beaches and he was walking into the trade winds as he moved from village to village, where he would conduct services for the faithful. The going depended very much on the wind and the tides. The grey sand was damp and firm after high tide but hot and soft when the tide was low. And the wind could be persistent.

'David walked alone on the last part of his trip from Magaubo towards his next destination at Darava village. He refused offers of company, possibly because he did not want to put anyone out, or because the villagers were reluctant, or maybe it was both. Anyway, it was a straight beach walk and he was young, fit, full of Christian zeal and he was, of course, a confident Australian.

'He never arrived.'

What would you do? How would you know where to begin to look?

Nick did the only thing that really works in wilder bush country, be it Africa or Papua New Guinea. He asked Soloi, his local 'go to' man, to find David.

Soloi did so with a combination of local knowledge and also, apparently, the supernatural. We rarely come across the supernatural in our investigations here in New Zealand, but it's stock-in-trade in the wilder parts of the world. Accompanied by two strapping young schoolboys, and assisted by the instructions he had divined from a vivid and compelling dream, Soloi made a beeline for Labu village, where the ferryman lived on the banks of the Bonua River. There on the far bank of the outlet to the sea, just as the dream had foretold, was a denuded and incomplete skeleton. Soloi and the two boys bore the remains back to Darava, enclosed in two pieces of a broken canoe secured with rope as a coffin. Then Soloi and the boys hastened back to carry the news to Dr Nick.

What was the terrible story of David's end?

There is no CIB out there to rush in and string plastic 'Police Emergency' tapes up around the scene. There is no homicide van filled with technology to sift for clues. There is no Environmental Science and Research (ESR) lab to conduct fine investigations and toxicology tests. There is only a district officer at remote Kupiano who represents the government, and all he would want was a written report in due course.

Nick's investigation was pretty good, I thought. Nick explained it to me.

'The Bonua River mouth has a one-and-a-half-kilometre backwater running behind the dunes where it meets the sea. You can't ferry across the mouth, which changes all the time and can be dangerous in some tides. You have to make your way on another track inland for a couple of kilometres until you are well behind the backwater. There, and only there, would there be a ferryman waiting to take you to Labu.

'David didn't know this, so he would have plunged on along the beach straight past the entrance to the inland track and come eventually to the river mouth.'

I could visualise this. There he would stand, looking in frustration across the wide river mouth. There would be no ferryman on either side that he could see, although he had been told there would be transport waiting. What could he do? Put yourself in his mind. What do you think he did?

Might he have stripped off to his underwear, left his luggage on the beach and swum across, intending to walk to the village and return with the ferryman to fetch his possessions? This looked a very plausible possibility to me.

'And guess what? Soloi found David's pack on the far beach exactly where we would expect it to be if that were the case. It contained three shirts, three singlets, three pairs of shorts, three pairs of socks, his shoes, his watch — but, tellingly, only two pairs of underwear.'

No man is going to swim a river and then walk into a village stark naked, is he? The numbers of clothes left behind tell the story of what he was thinking. David would have entered the river wearing that missing pair of underpants.

Now the back story was clear, I called Nick to talk about the possible causes of death.

'What did his body show?' I asked.

'I conducted the post-mortem, and I was particularly keen to get a positive identification,' Nick explained. 'I knew of a missionary who had disappeared without a trace and his wife had to wait seven years to be pronounced a widow. She wasn't free to remarry for those years, even if she'd had a mind to and of course she couldn't claim his insurance either. The identity was quite easy. He had a number of dental fillings, one of which I had put in, and their presence alone made it unlikely that the body was that of a Papuan. Later I had my records confirmed by David's dentist in Adelaide. I measured the skeleton from the ankle to the top of the skull at five foot ten. David was six foot tall.'

I nodded. 'That's about right once you add back the lost height of the muscles and tissues.'

'There was only a small scrap of scalp, but there were a couple of wavy black hairs just the colour and length that his were.'

'Were there any injuries?' With the tissues gone, only his bones were left to tell us his tale.

'Virtually all the soft tissue had been eaten by the fish. I could see their teeth marks even on the bones. The skeleton wasn't intact, though. Both feet, one arm and most of the fingers of the other hand were missing.'

I thought about that.

It had only been a week since David went missing. It is very unusual for a skeleton to fall apart in this way, especially after such a short period of time. The fibrous and elastic tissues around the joints are pretty tough and resilient and limbs won't peel away and disappear just like that. This sounded to me like an injury and not damage by fish or disintegration from decay.

'How do you think that happened, Nick?'

'I think it was a crocodile. There are many there in the Bonua River. That's why you need a permanent ferryman. The loss of his limbs looks to me like a crocodile.'

I agreed. 'Maybe even two or three smaller ones. He may have lost both his hands fighting off more than one. We had a family friend who was caught by two different crocodiles while fishing in the Zambezi River. One took his leg and the other came back for his arm. He fought them off each time, so they must have been quite small beasts. He eventually became the chief censor in Rhodesia and used to drive around in a modified VW Beetle.'

Straightforward drowning may also have been possible, but this did not fit quite so well because David was a strong swimmer. And why, then, would his limbs have been lost?

'I never heard what the district officer's findings eventually were, but I did have the honour of erecting a headstone over David's grave.'

It was an interesting story. Naturally, crocodiles and their activities are no part of our lives here in New Zealand, so I enjoyed hearing the intriguing story of David's death, which was so different from my usual daily diet of heart disease and diverticulitis. I thought then, in September 2017, that this would be the first and last crocodile story I'd come across in Palmerston North.

David Clarke. 1970. Requiescat in pace.

* * *

A lot of people hear news from Facebook these days. Almost unbelievably, more than half of all human conversations are now on social media. The news usually travels that way so much faster than by any other means. It was while we were sitting by our pool early one January morning in 2018, Elayne 'catching up' electronically with her tribe of people scattered across the world — as well as with those living only three doors down the road — that we heard the news.

'There's something here about Peter being bitten by a crocodile.' Elayne looked up at me.

'Where? How badly?' I asked.

Peter is Elayne's brother. He lives in Johannesburg, a big city that's not noted for its crocodile population. I imagined that perhaps Peter had got his finger too close to a hatchling held up by a keeper in a crocodile farm somewhere, and had suffered a bite as a consequence. It would be just like Pete to do that. Peter was a mining engineer until his recent retirement. He had spent his early life digging for gold ten thousand feet down on the reef, and in a lifelong teaching career, he has trained thousands of miners in the hard business of bringing the precious ores to the surface. Although he's in his seventies, he is very much what might be called a tearaway in New Zealand: always on the move, hiking and climbing, seeking out adventures that take him to the limits of danger. It's little wonder he sometimes manages to find himself in a spot of trouble.

'Doesn't say,' Elayne replied. 'Can't be too serious, then.'

I settled back and closed my eyes, basking in the summer sunshine. Most Facebook messages are trivial and deservedly ephemeral — information about big breakfasts eaten or stupendous sunsets seen. Nothing to see here.

Beside me, Elayne sighed.

'Suppose I'd better call and see.'

The Meat-Eaters

Peter and his family were on a bushveld holiday in Limpopo Province, right up in the top corner of South Africa hard by the borders with Mozambique and Zimbabwe and home to the Kruger National Park. It's still pretty wild up there, although not quite so wild as the old days when Sir Percy FitzPatrick wrote the well-known story *Jock of the Bushveld*, about his adventures with his Staffordshire bull terrier, Jock, set in the same part of the country. The plan was that they would meet up with Peter's son Graham and his wife, Jay, and their kids at a private holiday home on the banks of the Olifants River. It was Graham and Jay who had found the house, which looked idyllic: a happy family holiday home in the bush, with the river running by. It would sleep all nine of them, and it was cheap.

Peter's lot arrived first: Graham and Jay are both busy anaesthetists in Auckland, and they were taking a longer route to get there which would take in the sights of the Kruger National Park. Peter unloaded the mini-van and then headed out to see what was happening in the neighbourhood. He pulled on his swimmers, donned his prized, bright-orange hat and headed straight outside and down to the river bank, where there was a small swimming hole. His 18-year-old granddaughter, Savannah, joined him. It was 35 degrees — not too bad for an African summer. But it would soon get hotter as the sun climbed to its zenith.

'Look, Grandpa!' Savannah pointed.

A troop of vervet monkeys were chuntering for the trees. One was maimed, with only three limbs. Neither Pete nor Savannah thought anything much of that: there's always something trying to kill you in Africa. Maimed animals are pretty common.

The pool was cool and refreshing, although the temperature of most slackwater pools are in the low thirties in the low veld. On the far river bank, there was a homestay resort partly concealed by the bush. Here and there, there was evidence of other buildings. There was a rope swing tied to the branch of a tree on the river bank, so that kids could swing out high above the steep bank, let go and splash down into the running river, swim back to the bank and do it all again. Everything spoke of civilised holidays — sunburnt kids, refreshing splashing in the cool river and the aroma of barbecuing meat.

'Look!'

The rest of the family had by now come down to the river and they all looked where Peter was pointing.

There was a small island — more of a sandbar than a permanent feature — lying about 30 metres offshore, the river smoothly rippling past on either side. There was movement, a ruffling of sere, brown feathers. A naked, reptilian head craned up and cranked around to stare back at them. It was a vulture, but only one — not the flock you'd find clustered around the smorgasbord of a kill.

'He's worrying at something there,' Pete mused. 'Must be something dead over there. I wonder what it is?'

He paused for a moment, then made up his mind.

'Let's go across and have a look at the other side.'

Pete and Savannah walked upstream to where the bank sloped steeply but gave access to the water. They started across. It was only knee deep and it was cool. They were barefoot but the bottom was sandy and soft. The water was murky, though. Definitely murky.

'Pete! Come back! Come back now!' Lucy and Linda, his

wife and daughter, both shouted at the two. 'You don't know what's in there! Come back!'

Afterwards, Lucy said she had a premonition of what was about to happen. I've noticed over the years that womenfolk often object to the little adventures that men are prone to embark upon. But too often, it's not just idle: they seem sometimes to have a sense of fatal intuition. Men would probably be better off if they took the fears of women more seriously.

Pete and Savannah carried on wading to the far bank. It all seemed easy enough.

'Let's go back to that sandbank and maybe we can see what the vulture was after.'

The vulture flew off as they approached. The little strand had nothing to show, no steaming corpses to reward the expedition. While Savannah searched the sandy surface for a clue, Pete re-entered the water.

'I'm just going in here,' he called out, sliding down into a deeper channel gouged out by the current hard by the sandbank. The water here was waist deep, but the bottom was still soft and sandy.

Then Pete felt it beneath his foot, something hard, ribbed and crust-like. He knew straight away it was a crocodile's back, but there was just no time to react. The creature whipped around and caught his right leg in a grip like a vice. He was thrown from side to side, shaken the way a dog shakes a rat. Pete heard bones breaking, but strangely, he felt no pain. This isn't uncommon in situations like this. David Livingstone was attacked by a lion in 1844, leaving him with a badly mauled shoulder that pained him for the rest of his life. But he reported that at the time of the attack, he felt nothing but a strange euphoria. The body pours endorphins — naturally produced opioid hormones — into our bloodstream at times like this, which serve to numb the shock and pain.

Pete grabbed a breath whenever he could get his head above the water, but the croc never let go or so much as loosened its grip. Lucy and Linda looked on curiously from the bank. The animal was submerged in the murky water, and it was just so far outside their experience and what they expected, that they didn't suspect what was happening. Peter felt the need to explain.

'A crocodile's caught me!' he yelled.

'Are you joking?' Linda was incredulous. Pete is also a well-known prankster, so you always have to take what he says with a grain of salt.

'No, I'm bloody serious!' he screamed. 'It's got my leg!'

He knew how dire his situation was. He could still hear the damp, popping noise of breaking bone as the reptile re-asserted its grip. It seemed to go on and on. Surely there was nothing left to break?

Lucy and Linda were now screaming in full realisation of the horror. Where there's one crocodile, there'll surely be many more and close by, too. They're attracted by the sounds of struggle, doubtless out of an instinct to play the opportunist and steal some of the catch.

'Run!' they shouted at Savannah. 'Get out of there, quick!'

It was dangerous crossing the shallow channel back to the bank, but Savannah managed it and clambered sobbing up the steep, muddy slope to safety. Meanwhile, Peter was locked in a desperate struggle for survival. The crocodile threw him off balance again and again, trying to keep him under, but each time he would find a way to twist his body about and stand upright. All the same, it was only a matter of time before he weakened or the croc managed to hold him under for long enough. By now, he had a sense of how large it was. He reckoned it couldn't have been shorter than three metres from nose to tail: crocs this size generally weigh half a tonne. It was a massive mismatch.

By the grace of God, there were two rangers visiting another house nearby. They had seen Pete and Savannah wading across the river and were already phoning the different guesthouses to try to find someone there to get the pair out of the water pronto. They knew only too well what was living in that river. As soon as they heard Lucy and Linda screaming, they knew that their fears had been realised. They grabbed their rifles and some ammunition and rushed down to the river. They quickly found out from Pete that he was well and truly trapped.

Their arrival was timely. Peter took heart and renewed his fight.

'Don't try to open its mouth,' one ranger called out to him. 'You can't do it and it'll just grab your hand.'

The croc threw him again, and the twisting roll was accompanied by the sound of bones snapping or grating upon one another again. Yet again, Pete got his head clear of the surface and, knowing he had to do something, he reached forward and groped across the hard boss of the reptile's skull, looking for its eyes. He found the sockets and began pressing as hard as he could, trying to gouge out the eyes. But the croc simply squeezed its thick, leathery eyelids closed. All Pete could do was press on them as hard as he could.

There was an explosive crack and a splash. Then another, and another. Bullets began slapping into the water on either side as the rangers fired blindly into the river hoping to spook the crocodile. Ricochets howled off the surface, flying towards the bush on the far side. One shattered a resort window, but fortunately no-one was hit.

'Can you pick it up?' one of the rangers shouted. 'We can't see it from here. Pick it up so we can get a clear shot at it!'

Pete tried as hard as he could to heave some part of the creature above the surface, but he couldn't. The rangers kept shooting anyway, more in hope than expectation. One had to run back for more ammunition. The prospect of a rescue was rapidly slipping away from them. The croc was winning, edging Pete into deeper water. Pete experienced the sudden conviction that he was going to die. He wondered briefly what it felt like to drown. How long did it take?

Just as he tried to rally, the crocodile changed tactics again. As Pete went underwater, disorientated, he felt a huge blow on his chest. A wave of weakness flowed down his arms. The conviction that he was lost returned.

Crocodiles are an evolutionary success story. They've been around, virtually unchanged, since the time of the dinosaurs, thanks to a suite of tricks they have acquired that have served them well for millions of years. They will shake their victim from side to side, just as this one had shaken Pete. Of course, everyone knows their 'death roll', where they will latch onto you and roll over, lying with you in a loving embrace on the river bottom as the bubbles burst from your throat and the dark water floods into your lungs. But they also have a cat-like tactic where they bring up the wicked claws on their hind feet and kick and tear at your belly and chest.

The Meat-Eaters

That's what the beast did to Pete, inflicting horrific injuries. Both of his shoulders were shattered and his wrists fractured. Raking talons broke his breastbone and injured his heart. Those were the main injuries: never mind the lacerations, gouges and bruises.

Somehow, Pete summoned the strength to have another go at its eyeballs. Perhaps it was this. Perhaps it was because the crocodile had exhausted the energy budget for this fight — they have huge levels of lactic acid in their blood, the chemical that settles in your muscles and tells you that it is time to stop exercising. Perhaps it just ran out of steam. Or because it had briefly emerged in executing its terrible ripping assault on Pete, one of the bullets finally found its mark. Whatever it was, the creature suddenly released Pete and glided away.

Pete managed to drag himself to the sandbank. He called out to the rangers that it had let him go.

Without a second's hesitation, even knowing the risk of another attack was very high, the ranger named Paul rushed into the river, seized Pete and carried him back to the shore. It was an act of selfless bravery. It had been 15 long minutes since the onslaught began. A quarter of an hour in the water wrestling with a three-metre crocodile must be some sort of record, although it's not one you'd want to try to beat.

Pete was a dreadful sight. He was alive, but it wasn't certain for how much longer. His leg was smashed with spicules of muddied bone and mushed flesh, crushed and fouled by the effluvium from the dinosaur's fangs. Blood coursed freely from his many wounds. His arms and shoulders were misshapen, fractured and dislocated. He needed emergency surgery and advanced intensive care from a sophisticated hospital and he needed it right away. But here he was, way out in the wilds, far, far from that sort of help.

He drifted into unconsciousness.

There was no rescue helicopter service. An ambulance was called. It had to come from Hoedspruit, the closest town about 30 minutes away. In the meantime, the family and the rangers did what they could out there in the bush — not that there was much they could offer beyond basic first aid. A paramedic arrived and continued the stabilisation, but he had no equipment to speak of, not so much as a saline drip to mitigate the rampant blood loss.

The ambulance arrived. They took one look at Pete's injuries and shook their heads.

'No use going to Hoedspruit. There's no-one at the hospital who can help him with these injuries. He will have to go to Polokwane.'

Polokwane is an hour and a half's drive on winding, rugged dirt roads. It's easy to get lost if you're not familiar with the way, but that wasn't the immediate problem.

'We haven't got enough petrol to get there.' The driver shrugged. 'We'll have to fill up on the way.'

Pete was loaded into the back of the ambulance. He lay on a steel stretcher but there was no pillow. The only painkillers were Panadol tablets. But at least he was heading towards the help he needed if he was to see the sunrise the next day, let alone any other.

The ambulance lurched over the rough roads as the tropical sun reached its zenith. The temperature in the cabin reached 40 degrees. They pulled into a service station and the driver began to fill the tank. A middle-aged man was filling up the tank of his car at an adjacent pump while his family waited inside. It's not often you see an ambulance filling up at a garage, even in Africa.

'What are you doing here?' the man asked. 'Where are you going?'

The ambulance driver told him the story.

'Let me have a look. I'm a doctor.'

The man climbed in the back and looked down in horror and disbelief. The victim was his father.

Graham had stopped at the same garage to fill up on his way to the guesthouse by the river. There was nothing for it but to climb in and do what he could. Graham is an anaesthetist and a very experienced ICU doctor but, of course, he could do little without staff and equipment and oxygen and blood. Take any modern doctor away from the technology-rich, well-staffed environments in which they're accustomed to operate and most will be little more use to you than any other basically trained first-aider.

Peter was still with them as they reached Polokwane Hospital, just. Graham was relieved to deliver his dad to a facility that had resuscitation, blood, pain relief and theatres where the injuries could be cleaned. He was impressed with the way the staff immediately swung into action. It plainly wasn't their first crocodile attack. All the same, he knew that Pete stood only a slim chance unless he could get the very best treatment, better than a provincial hospital could reasonably be expected to provide. Graham had done his medical training at Witwatersrand University in Johannesburg and he knew there was an outstanding trauma unit at Milpark Hospital. That's where Nelson Mandela was sent for treatment.

Milpark was four hours away by road and Pete's 'Golden Hour' had long since run its course. A helicopter seemed his only chance. Money was no problem — Pete had the finest medical insurance cover from his years of mining with the Anglo American Corporation — but there was a typically African hurdle to surmount before a chopper would be dispatched. Graham had to get a medical assessment of Pete's chances of survival. Only if he was certified with a bolter's chance would the chopper take to the air. It seems brutal to New Zealanders, for whom the rescue helicopter service is always there on call, but there is some logic in a land where distances are vast and medical services are spread very thinly.

Even once he'd been admitted to the intensive care unit in Johannesburg, Peter's life was hanging in the balance. Elayne and I followed as best we could, each ping of her phone bringing another snippet of news. For the first few hours, the news was not good.

'His heart is damaged and is failing,' Graham reported. 'He is on inotropic drugs which are barely keeping his blood pressure up. His blood bicarbonate is falling to dangerously low levels. His kidneys have failed …'

We were preparing ourselves for the ping that would bring the news that the worst had happened.

'The sepsis to come will be the critical factor,' Graham reported.

'It will be the leg that is the problem,' I said to Elayne. 'It will be pouring bacteria and toxins into his system and those will be overwhelming.'

Sure enough, the news came through that Pete's leg had been amputated. It is not a light decision to sacrifice a leg, but Pete was in no state to be consulted. Not that there was any doubt: it was gangrenous, crushed and fouled by the

The Meat-Eaters

animal's filthy fangs. It was rapidly and surely killing Pete as he lay there.

'It was a relief to have it gone,' Graham texted. 'We do not regret the decision. It was stinking and unsalvageable. His blood biochemistry has since turned and is going the right way now. We now have to get through the inevitable pneumonia.'

As Pete stabilised, Graham found the time and mental space to pay tribute to Paul, the ranger who had pulled Pete from the river. 'However this all ends, we shall forever be grateful for the incredible bravery of the ranger who went into the water at such personal risk to save Dad.'

The journey back was slow and long but the tough miner fought in his ICU bed every bit as hard as he had fought in that river. He regained consciousness. Then he was declared out of danger. Soon he was even talking about prosthetic limbs. From that point on, his recovery was steady. Within a year of losing his leg to the crocodile, he had rejoined the group with whom he regularly does a five-kilometre park run on a Saturday morning, and had met a personal goal of swimming a mile. His story is a testament to human courage and endurance.

When he tells the story, Pete always calls the crocodile 'he', but the odds are that this was a female. In Southern Africa, the females stay put in a trance-like state for the three months up to Christmas, guarding their nests. They do not eat at all during that time so naturally they head out afterwards starving and empty-bellied for a catch-up feed. The busiest time for attacks is in the first three months of the new year, and many of these are, of course, due to the famished females.

But how the hell did this crocodile come to be lying up amongst the holiday homes, close by a children's rope swing into the river? I wondered. I knew that they could travel huge distances overland. And as I read around the subject, I decided that, quite possibly, this one came from a crocodile farm. In 2013, the Limpopo River burst its banks and crocodile farmer Johan Boshoff had to open the gates on the Rakwena Crocodile Farm to release the surging flood tide. Fifteen thousand crocodiles escaped and fewer than half were recaptured. One travelled an unbelievable 120 kilometres and was found on the rugby field of a high school in Musina.

Could it be that the remainder spread out through the rivers and across the Limpopo bush district, travelling overland where necessary? They couldn't all stay in the Limpopo River, which was already chock-full of crocs. There wouldn't be enough game to go around, and the pressure to move out to the south and the east to seek new rivers and waterways would be immense. The same pressures for new territory are pushing the saltwater crocodiles in Australia inland and more and more into human settlements.

Apparently there had even been a warning issued in relation to the Olifants River. Only a couple of months before Pete was attacked, Lt-Col Ngoepe from the Limpopo police told locals that: 'There has been a mushrooming of crocodiles in the Olifants River, so be careful crossing the river.' How exactly one is careful sharing a waterway with a 500-kilogram predator, I'm not sure.

* * *

The Meat-Eaters

New Zealanders can be thankful that we don't have those ancient and terrible crocodiles. But we do have other, equally ancient meat-eaters that can assault you unexpectedly and they are every bit as horrible and implacable as any African ambush predator.

I was walking through the lab when Mike Young came in wearing his scrubs. Mike was a young, newly qualified general surgeon in those days, but highly competent and enthusiastic. There was a sheen of sweat on his forehead, so he must have been busy plying his trade.

'What's up, Mike?'

'Just done a hindquarter. My first.'

A hindquarter amputation. Wow! My first, too.

There weren't many reasons to do them. The surgeon has to amputate the leg and half of the pelvis, splitting the pubis down the middle and detaching the sacrum from the pelvic bone as well as all the major muscles. It is a horrible and mutilating operation which is usually reserved for big cancers of the pelvis.

But I knew it wasn't a cancer. If it were, I would have seen a biopsy and there would have been much discussion before the decision was taken to perform such major surgery. This had evidently come out of the blue.

'What's happened?'

Mike shook his head and rubbed his brow.

'Necrotising fasciitis.'

Necrotising fasciitis. Oh God, no!

The newspapers, always with an eye to sensation, had christened this bacterium 'the flesh-eating bug', and I've always thought that was a better name than the technical one, necrotising fasciitis.

'What's happened? Is the patient dead?'

Why else would Mike be here? I wondered. The diagnosis of this disease was always so obvious at first sight of the patient that a pathologist wasn't needed to give guidance. I was invariably called in at the death to do an autopsy. Although these were natural deaths, they are so fast, so ghastly and unbelievable that doctors are often reluctant to accept it and unwilling to sign a death certificate. It's as though, having been unable to do more for the patient in life, there's a sense that more should be done after death, such as an autopsy and a coronial inquiry.

'No, not dead. In ICU. She's only 18.' He looked stunned. 'The orthopaedic surgeons had admitted her after her leg became painful and swollen. They called me pretty quickly because it was getting worse.'

He shook his head again.

'Boy, it was moving fast. The skin was bubbling and getting darker as you watched. By the time I'd got theatre organised, it had reached her groin and she was pretty toxic. I had no choice but to cut it all out and that meant a hindquarter. I took it off as quickly as I could and got her out of there and into ICU. It's not looking good, so I'm just giving you a heads-up.'

I nodded. In those days, a death within 24 hours of surgery was always referred to the coroner and an autopsy carried out. I guess an autopsy was a good check and balance in earlier eras of surgery and the habit had persisted. Autopsies are no longer automatic after a surgical death today, as so much more is known and already documented during the operation.

'I suppose she's in septic shock?'

Mike nodded sombrely. The heart and circulation went into collapse under the toxic assault of the meat-eating bugs and that was really hard to treat. Antibiotics alone were not enough and a cocktail of potent drugs was needed to keep the heart pumping and the brain and kidneys supplied with enough oxygenated blood to stay alive and functioning.

It was always touch and go. The night would be decisive.

Ian, the mortuary assistant, called before eight.

'Good morning, Doctor. Your customer is ready for you.'

I hated him calling them customers, but it was ingrained. They are my patients — not customers, not cases and certainly not clients, as modern hospital management would have us call them.

Her name was Eva Burnell. She had not survived the night. Despite everything humanly possible having been done, the bacterial brew proved overwhelming, and in the small hours of the morning her heart finally stopped beating. Her autopsy was typical of patients from Intensive Care. There was a plethora of lines and tubes to examine and remove, from tracheal tubes to arterial lines, catheters and drains from the massive surgical wounds. All were checked and documented. All were confirmed to be correctly placed and functional.

Eva was a pretty redhead, at peace now her ordeal had passed. There was nothing at all to find in my autopsy. That was not unexpected. The diseased leg was off and death was due to septicaemia and that is usually quite invisible at autopsy. The hidden bugs may be riddling the bloodstream and I could capture samples of them and grow the hateful beasts in an agar plate in the microbiology laboratory, but I couldn't see them here on the table.

Her organs were those expected of a healthy young woman with nothing to show for the wash of bacterial poisons in which they had finally foundered.

'What is this flesh-eating bug, Doc?' The hospital policeman, Peter Kos, had come down to the mortuary with the paperwork.

'It's often not one bug, but several species. A bit of a mixed bag of species, like a whitebait catch, really. When you grow them, there are staphylococci and streptococci as well as common gut bacteria. All the usual bugs that you and I both have living all around us and not causing any trouble. But sometimes they get into a gang and for some reason they go berserk. They attack the blood vessels and destroy the deeper fat and tissue. The whole lot just goes gangrenous and it spreads like an Aussie bush fire.

'I was once sent a young mother who was hit on the shoulder by a flying fox in a playground. She got pretty bad bruising and swelling from the blow. There must also have been a break in the skin, because she got the flesh-eating bug and died pretty quickly. The Accident Compensation Corporation refused to accept it was an accident, saying it was an infectious disease. I had to write a report telling them that, although the accident may have seemed trivial at the time, the massive infection should not obscure that it was the accident that was the cause of death. Fortunately, they accepted my opinion and paid the family out. It was only a few thousand for the funeral in the end.'

I had Eva's amputated leg and half pelvis brought out of the mortuary fridge and examined it. Now here there was pathology to be seen. The skin was blotched with purple and red patterns on which were the raised pocks of disfiguring, flaccid blisters. The deep thigh and calf muscles were an unhealthy devitalised grey, their death and destruction already quite advanced. The fat beneath the skin was a dirty lemon colour and was smearing and liquefying as I touched it.

I examined the skin surface minutely. Where had this started? I knew that, in young people, the disease started with a slight injury through which the meat-eaters penetrated the defences of the skin.

'Ah, look! What's this?' I was looking at the sole of the foot. There in the centre of the ball of the foot was a roughened blemish. It was an injury site.

'This is it. This must be the entry point.'

Peter looked with interest. 'What's caused that, do you think?'

'I'm not sure. It's an odd place to have stood on something. Looks more like a minor operation site to me.' I looked up. 'Can you find out if Eva had had any minor surgery? Check with her GP.'

Peter nodded. I took a biopsy of the site to examine under the microscope. It turned out to be a small wart, a verruca of the foot. These warts often infest the soles of the feet of young adults, and I can tell you from personal experience that they're damned uncomfortable. They feel so much like you've got a thorn or piece of glass in your foot that GPs often cut them out thinking there's something in there.

We found out that Eva apparently had thought she had a splinter of glass and had dug around in there without success. She had then gone to her GP who agreed and also had a fruitless dig. That was surely the point of entry for the bugs. The GP prescribed her Voltaren as a painkiller, though her pain wasn't really too bad.

Voltaren is a great painkiller. It's dished out like lollies at the Christmas parade for all sorts of things and it's generally quite safe. But not always. The flesh-eating bug has increased its attacks on Kiwis threefold since 1990 and one of the reasons is reckoned to be a huge increase in the use of non-steroidal anti-inflammatory drugs such as Voltaren. What the drugs have to do with this is not really understood, but nonetheless it is surprising how often they pitch up in the back story of patients with necrotising fasciitis.

Who can say what effect the Voltaren had on Eva? Maybe it played some part in letting the bug in; maybe it masked the symptoms until too late. No-one really knows how it acts, but the written evidence is convincing that Voltaren is at least an accessory to the crime.

And so the sad autopsy was done and the cause of death recorded: death was due to septic shock from necrotising fasciitis. A natural death from a natural disease caused by creatures sharing the world with us.

Not so very different from a crocodile attack, really.

Eva Burnell. October 1993. Requiescat in pace.

CHAPTER 6

Line of Duty

'The entry wound is here' — Bruce Lockett pointed at the jagged-edged cavity — 'just over the back of the eighth rib on his right side.' The detectives of the homicide squad craned forward to look. All homicide autopsies have an air of gravity, but today was very different. There was an edge of anger here, too.

'The bullet has entered horizontally so both he and the shooter must have been standing. It's smashed the back of the eighth and ninth ribs, before taking out the ninth vertebra and then doing the same to the back of the eighth rib on the left side of his back.'

'So not a full-frontal shot? Could he have been running towards the shooter?'

Bruce shook his head. 'I think this shows he must have been side-on to the rifle when hit.'

'Was that the cause of death?' Ross Grantham's face was working to control an emotion.

Bruce nodded. 'The spinal cord is damaged, too, over a considerable length, and the cerebrospinal fluid is heavily bloodstained, so spinal shock is the major cause. But there are also shock-wave cavities punched out on the back of the lungs on both sides. They're pretty serious, too. The one on the right is at least eight centimetres across.'

Spinal shock. I agreed that was the cause.

People often ask how a bullet kills you when it doesn't do something obvious like blow your heart or brain to bits. No-one really knows for sure, but it seems the massive shock waves just pile on a tidal wave of nervous signals to the brain, or more scientifically, to the reticular activating system, which more or less blows the fuse, and life just shuts down, pretty well instantaneously.

It was lunchtime on Saturday, 6 July 2002, and for a weekend the mortuary was in an uncharacteristic frenzy of activity. It had all started 24 hours before.

'Reports are just coming in that a policeman has been shot and killed this afternoon in the rural Manawatu near the town of Rongotea. We will bring you updates as they come to light.'

'Not us again!' I heard the news late on Friday afternoon as I was passing through Shannon on my way back from Wellington. That was my first thought and my heart sank. My second was: 'I wonder who it is?' Afterwards, I was embarrassed, as this should have been my first thought. I knew so many of the local officers and it made this news very personal.

'Who's on call?' I next wondered. Bruce Lockett was in the lab so I knew we would be able to respond immediately when called.

As soon as I got to Palmerston North that evening, I went straight up to the lab. Bruce was still there.

'Who is it?' I couldn't contain myself. 'What happened?'

Bruce shook his head sorrowfully. 'It's Duncan. Duncan Taylor. And Jeanette.'

'Oh no! Jeanette as well? I thought the radio said there was only one?' Of course, Jeanette would be there. She and Duncan were partners.

'She's been hit. She's okay. She's here in the hospital.'

It seemed scarcely possible. My mind flicked back to the case of the skeletonised man. Wasn't that only six months ago?

Duncan. Oh no, not that gentle giant of a man.

Ross Grantham, Jeanette's boss, arrived unannounced in the lab with an entourage of CIB detectives. He had some photographs to show me. They were of Jeanette's wound.

'What do you think?'

Bruce and I examined the injury critically. 'A burst type wound. A through-and-through shot with shock waves bursting the skin above the track. Or a peripheral glancing hit ploughing a furrow. Either could make that sort of injury.'

Ross nodded. 'That's what we thought. It fits with what happened.'

We soon heard the whole story. Bruce had carried out the autopsy on Duncan on Saturday as soon as Duncan's body could be retrieved from the scene of the killing. As for any murder, we needed to meticulously document evidence for court.

'The perpetrator is Daniel Luff who is just a boy, really, only 17 years old.' Ross shook his head sadly. Ross was a tough cop. He was obviously moved by the pointlessness of

Duncan's death but I also wondered whether he wasn't also sickened by the tragedy of Daniel's youth.

'He had a restraining order in place preventing him from seeing or visiting his ex-girlfriend, Stephanie. Stephanie lives on the farm there on Taipo Road with her parents, Robert and Christine Cocker. Dad is a dairy farmer. She had gone out with Luff over the past year but they broke up in May. He took it bloody hard. Wouldn't leave her alone or let it go. Eventually it was the parents who took out the restraining order.'

'Is he obsessional or just love-sick?' I asked. Young men, I know, go off their food when in love and then they really don't think things through very rationally, do they? But not every love-sick young man shoots police officers.

Ross shrugged. He didn't know. Like myself, I'm not sure Ross's strong point was psychology. That's why I'm a pathologist, of course, and he's a detective.

'He's pretty bright. He rebuilds Land Rovers. Apparently he has four in bits lying around their yard. He was in one when Duncan and Jeanette saw him. They knew him well, partly because of the restraining order, but also because there had been a pile of petty thieving around the area and he was a person of interest to us.'

Duncan and Jeanette were surprised to see Daniel passing by as he was supposed to be visiting his grandfather in Samoa, a holiday that had been arranged to get some physical distance between him and Stephanie. They decided to call on the Cocker family and warn them he was back in town.

The family were just sitting down to lunch. Duncan and Jeanette were outside talking to Robert Cocker when Daniel roared past the house in his dark-green Land Rover without stopping. The Feilding detectives decided to give chase to talk to Daniel and remind him to keep well away from the farm. Daniel saw the flashing police lights and something in his mind snapped. He pulled over at once and as the police car passed he grinned through the side window at Jeanette.

He didn't wait for them. He whipped his Land Rover around and sped back towards the Cockers' farm, where he skidded to a halt and leapt out, pulling a loaded Voere .270 rifle out from behind him and rushing inside.

Things now had their own momentum.

Duncan and Jeanette drew up and, unarmed, ran towards the farmhouse. Duncan was in the lead. He saw Daniel raise his rifle and point it. He pivoted away towards his left screaming at Jeanette.

'Run! He's got a gun!'

Daniel shot him in the right side of his chest as he was turning away. Duncan fell to the ground, killed instantly.

Jeanette saw Daniel grin at her again as he swung the rifle on her. Jeanette is small and fast, very fast. She ran away, zig-zagging. Three shots boomed after her. One winged her but she kept going. Another screamed past her head, just missing her. Daniel was a very good shot but her size, speed and evasive action made her a difficult target. She managed to get into a ditch and make her way along to a neighbour's house about 500 metres away, where she raised the alarm.

Meanwhile, back at the farm, the situation was tense. Robert Cocker had seen Duncan shot and fall dead, and he rushed in to protect his family. Stephanie was hidden in a cupboard and the Cockers managed to barricade themselves in a room.

Daniel waited quietly, his rifle loaded, watching for any movement. He didn't have to wait long.

The Armed Offenders Squad arrived and a five-hour siege began. The access roads were sealed. No-one could get in or out, or even close. A telephone link was made with Daniel and a negotiator began his patient persuasion. Stephanie managed to escape the house through a window and ran to a neighbour's for help. She drew a plan of the house with Daniel's location marked. The problem was that her parents were still trapped inside.

Meanwhile, Daniel's mother, Tracey, somehow heard the news and she did what any mother would do: she rushed to the aid of her son. Tracey came to the road block, tried to drive around it, and when that failed, she left her car with the engine running, the lights on and door open, and started running towards the farmhouse. She was stopped and taken back. After regaining her composure, she helped out by trying to cajole Daniel to surrender.

Daniel told the police that they need not bother trying to evacuate Duncan, as he was definitely dead. He warned them not to try anything, as he was an expert shot. To prove his point, he shot a fence post just beside a detective's head, the round blowing it apart. Doug Brew was in charge of the siege. He kept everyone calm and out of the line of fire while Daniel was persuaded to give himself up. No-one wanted another death, least of all that of a 17-year-old, no matter how terrible the thing that he had done.

Things broke when the Cockers followed Stephanie's escape route out and also got clear away. Two tear-gas canisters were then fired into the house and in went the dogs. It was soon over, thank God, although for us, it was just beginning, and the agony of shattered lives would last forever for the families.

Why did he do it?

Daniel had been born to drug-addicted parents. His father was an active user and had a string of convictions, but was largely absent from Daniel's life. His mother, Tracey, had addiction issues of her own, and Daniel was removed and shipped from pillar to post in the state system until he was eight, when Tracey had got her own life together enough to take him back and to try to repair some of the damage done. She seems to have made some headway. He was reckoned a good student at Awatapu College, despite the disjointed beginning his education had got off to in over a dozen schools. His teachers considered him to be thoughtful and dedicated. Oddly, he was a skilled locksmith and collector of padlocks. Less oddly, he was mad keen on hunting, as so many young men are. I know I was in my youth back in Africa, so I wouldn't hold that against him. The standard explanation for the tragedy would be to point to an obsessional personality, citing the fixation with Land Rovers, locks and guns. He was described, inevitably as it seems, as a 'loner' by some. The psychologists duly decided that the lack of insight into his offending that they perceived was 'more than the "unreasonable detachment" of an emotionally vulnerable teen. It is more likely an inborn personality disorder and the shooting of Duncan not so much a crime of passion as the detached behaviour of a cold-blooded killer.'

Daniel was sentenced to life imprisonment with 17 years' minimum non-parole for Duncan's murder and for the attempted murder of Jeanette. If the psychologists were truly right and Daniel had some innate flaw, then surely there would be no way back, no hope of a change in prison, no possibility of redemption?

The judge, while reflecting the seriousness of his offending with the non-parole period, seems to have thought there was some prospect of rehabilitation, otherwise why not preventive detention for life? Daniel's teachers, or some of them, thought he was far from a lost cause. I found out later that Duncan, too, had made Daniel a kind of personal project, seeing in him the potential for better things.

And perhaps there is a spark of hope, after all. In an article about him and his crime in *North & South* magazine in 2018, Daniel described his imprisonment in Paremoremo as being deserved '— all for poor decisions motivated by a mix of immaturity, self-centredness, institutionalisation and boredom'. This seems insightful. He certainly felt remorse, and described his anguish as he told his mother: 'He [Duncan] had a baby, Ma. He had a baby!' Before those terrible events, Daniel had bumped into Duncan, his partner and their baby in a café. Many murderers lack empathy, and are incapable of fully appreciating the harm they have done as a consequence. I don't think Daniel falls into that category.

It's nearly 18 years since the murder. The 17-year-old killer has turned into a 35-year-old man while in prison. And it seems the years weren't entirely consumed by the locusts: while in prison, Daniel finished school, enrolled at university and graduated with a Bachelor of Arts with Honours. He has since started a PhD investigating aspects of the rehabilitation process for offenders. His first bid for an early release was declined by the Parole Board, but he will face them again in May 2021. Whatever the eventual outcome of his appeal, we have to keep faith in the chance of ultimate redemption for all of us, for that is what makes society civilised rather than blindly retributive. Otherwise, what's the point? Even more lives are wasted, and tragedy is heaped on tragedy.

*Duncan Taylor, New Zealand Police. 6 July 2002.
Requiescat in pace.*

* * *

Everyone loves Christmas. Parties and presents, family, food and festivities. Not a great time for murder, if ever there *was* a great time for a murder.

A Christmas party, no different from many others over the years and like thousands of other such gatherings happening all around the country, was taking place at the Rongotea Tavern on 16 December 2001. Amongst the revellers were Paul Allen and Helen Johns, who were relatively recent partners. They had a good time and left early in the evening for their farm on Hammond Street.

Douglas Arthur Thompson followed them back, Ross Grantham told me.

'He says he went round to take them a Christmas card.'

I looked at Ross incredulously. Had I heard that right?

'Of course he did,' he said, catching my look. 'As one does. More to the point, he took along his rifle as well as the card.'

Paul was the new man on Helen's scene. Thompson was Helen's estranged ex-partner. Apparently the parting had been an unpleasant and acrimonious business.

'A rifle? Now that's a very festive idea! And what happened?'

'Paul Allen is dead outside the front door on the lawn. Gunshot wound. We're not sure where he was hit. Helen

Johns managed to get clear and inside where she called 111 at 8:42 p.m. She was kept on the line talking to the operator until 9.18, when she went offline. So we got the first part of the story. It took a while to get the Armed Offenders Squad out there. By the time they'd secured the area and got inside it was 10.15 p.m.'

I was opening my mouth to ask the obvious question, but Ross shook his head grimly.

'Helen was dead. Also a gunshot wound.'

I guess you hope the police will reach you pretty pronto when you're under the gun, as it were, but it wasn't possible, this time. The press were asking questions. Where was the Armed Offenders Squad when Helen was talking to the 111 operator all that time? Did they react too slowly? And even if they couldn't have got there in time to prevent her shooting, surely the AOS could have reached her in time to save her? Her injuries were said to have been survivable if only help had reached her sooner. It left a nasty taste in an already nasty tragedy.

Never mind that there were reasonable explanations for the delays. Back then, Palmerston North had only a part-time Armed Offenders Squad. When they were called out, they had to rush down to the station, hastily pull on their bulletproof vests, helmets and radio gear as well as draw their weapons and ammunition. And, of course, they had to have a briefing about what the hell was going on, who was their target and how well they were armed. That all has to happen before they set off. Then it's still a good 25 kilometres out to Rongotea and further on still from there to the Hammond Street farm.

By the time they arrived, it was getting late. The farm was in darkness and it had started to rain, although Paul Allen's body was visible lying close to the front door. The critical question nagging at everyone's mind now was: Where was Thompson?

The outhouses first needed to be checked and secured. They were pretty well spread out. By the time that was done, it had been over half an hour since Helen was last heard from.

At last, the AOS went into the house, tense and alert. They quickly found Helen, and it was clear that they were too late.

That was the scene I found the next morning when I arrived with a couple of registrars. These were the pathologists in training and they were there to learn how to examine a murder scene in order to make the fatal events clear and to determine the method of the murder. The idea is that out of chaos and confusion, our analysis should produce order, answers and clarity.

Lying on a patch of lawn by the driveway was the body of a well-muscled, swarthy young man wearing dark-green shorts. He had an exuberant dark moustache and there was fresh abrasions on his upper lip. One of the registrars pointed at the injury.

'Someone's just clocked him there.'

'Shush!' I warned him.

I looked around hurriedly. Fortunately, no-one had heard.

My young colleague was absolutely right: that is exactly what it looked like. But we have to be cautious during any murder investigation. Police follow you everywhere writing down every word you say. What may be idle speculation at the time will get dredged up by a defence lawyer later in court and represented as an absolute fact. Or worse, if your first impression is at odds with the more considered opinion you derive from careful examination, you can bet you'll be charged with being unsure, of not knowing your own mind, of giving unreliable evidence. It's infuriating, but alas! That's how our adversarial system works.

'The golden rule is to say nothing until we've seen everything,' I admonished him.

He was unabashed.

'We're wasting our time hanging around here. Why can't we just go inside now?'

I sighed. This registrar was never going to make a forensic pathologist, I decided. My instincts were proven quite right. In future years, he was to become a highly regarded specialist in the pathology of skin rashes and diseases in Australia. But he was too impetuous for the meticulous, methodical work demanded at a crime scene.

I examined Paul Allen first. He was shot twice. He must have been on his feet for the first. Like Duncan Taylor, the indications were that he was turning away from the man with the rifle when it was fired. Perhaps he was turning to run. Who can tell?

That bullet went horizontally into the right side of his chest and punched through the muscles to the left side. It did nothing serious.

My impression was that he was then struck in the face, damaging his lip, but whether the injury was inflicted with the butt of the gun or a fist, I couldn't tell. He would already have been stunned by the shock of the first bullet, but it would have been the blow to the face that knocked him to the ground for sure.

The second bullet was the fatal one. This was in the front of the chest just to the left of the breastbone and the indications were that it was fired from close range, very close. There was a dark stain at the wound's edges.

I pointed this out to my registrars.

'Look. That's a burn from the muzzle flash. It's different from the powder stippling you get when the shot is fired from further away. You get this burning when the range is close or actually at point-blank.'

Later, in the mortuary, we had the opportunity to study this wound more closely.

'The black rim around the entry wound doesn't wipe off as soot would,' I explained, and examined the bluish-black staining with a magnifying glass. 'It's not a speckled abrasion from gunpowder stippling,' I added. 'It's definitely a muzzle burn. That's point-blank range.'

It wasn't just a first time for the registrars, who were seeing their first death by gunshot wound. This case was a first for me, too, as it was the first time I had the opportunity to have a CAT scan done on the body. This uses computer imaging (hence the name: computer assisted tomography) to collate the results of dozens of passes by a scanner into a single, virtual picture, like building up a 3D puzzle layer by thin layer. The results were amazing. The bullet track could be seen at once without the need for hours spent in tedious dissection.

Sean Gallagher, the radiologist, talked us through it, pointing at the glowing screen.

'The track is lined by air which makes it easy to see. It's hit the heart for certain.' He frowned, peering closely. 'Not sure where, exactly, but it's also punctured the left lung, which has collapsed. The chest is full of blood. Together, that heart and the lung injury, that's what killed him.'

'Thanks, Sean. That's really helpful. We'll bring the other victim down in a couple of hours, if that's okay?'

'Sure. By the way, the bullet deflected off the bottom of the eighth rib and is in the back of the chest wall.'

And so it proved.

As the CIB gathered around me at the dissecting bench, I used the large rib secateurs to shear the ribs on either side of the breastbone. I lifted the breastbone off with the wet noise of the tearing of soft tissue. In this way, I could open the chest while keeping the bullet entrance wound intact. Nearly half of Paul's blood was lying free in his chest cavity. That wasn't surprising.

'The bullet's made a huge hole, two to four centimetres across, going straight through both sides of the heart.'

'Where was it fired from?'

Of course, Ross was immediately on to the most important question. I thought carefully before answering, assembling all of my observations into a single picture of what had happened — a kind of mental equivalent of the CAT scan.

'From the front, certainly. At point-blank or just off the skin, highly probably. From Paul's right side pointing down to his left, likely. It looks to me as if Paul was lying on the ground with the rifle pointing downwards over his right shoulder aimed directly at the left side of the chest.'

I enacted the scene over his body for clarity.

With Sean's CAT scan providing pinpoint guidance, I easily found the .22 calibre bullet and into a pottle it went for the forensic scientists to mull over.

By the time we had painted a picture of the execution-style murder of Paul Allen, the day was already drawing to a weary close. But now it was Helen's turn. We needed to see if we could determine what had happened to her after her frantic 111 call was cut off.

I had already spent a long time inside the house, crouched over Helen examining her position and poring over the surrounding scene. As the picture grew, I was appalled at the awfulness of it. On the scale of things, the injuries weren't that gross or grotesque. It's just that I kept imagining that poor woman hiding, terrified, in her own house, the cool voice of the 111 operator on the other end of the line her only link to the prospect of rescue. Helen knew what had happened to Paul. At the very least, she had heard the gunshots. She may even have witnessed the murder unfold. The call lasted 36 minutes.

Then what?

There was a jagged laceration over the pulp of the right middle finger. This, I decided, must have happened when Thompson arrived and pointed the rifle at her. She had grasped the muzzle, and it had been forcibly pulled away from her through her tightly closed hand. The little metal tang of the foresight had ripped her finger.

From then on, events followed roughly the same course as Paul's killing. There was a similar burst wound to the upper lip, certainly a hard physical blow and enough to knock her to the floor. She had been killed by a single shot. The bullet tore from top to bottom through the right lung down through the vena cava, which usually carries the lion's share of all our circulating blood, and ploughed into her liver. Most tellingly, it also sliced open the right atrium, the thin-walled upper chamber on top of the heart, on its way through.

'The atrium is effectively a bag of blood,' I explained to the detectives. 'And the contents have poured into the pericardium, the sac around the heart, creating a pericardial tamponade.'

'What does that do?'

'The sac fills up and literally squeezes the heart to death. The pressure just stops it beating. It takes minutes at the most.'

I thought Helen, like Paul, had been lying on the floor when shot by someone standing over her. The burnt skin around the wound indicated a close discharge, no more than a centimetre or two away, but probably a lot closer.

My mind turned to the press commentary on the delay in getting help to Helen. I knew the police were vexed by the media's uninformed assertions. Police response times are for them to justify, but I could at least give an opinion on whether Helen might have survived if they had reached her sooner. I asked Bruce Rhind, the senior general surgeon on call, to come down to the mortuary and give his opinion.

I showed Bruce the extent of the wound and the hole punctured in the atrium.

'The hole is big and the tamponade would be sudden and overwhelming. There was 250 millilitres of blood in the pericardial sac and nearly another litre sloshing around freely inside the chest. I don't think she could have survived that.'

Bruce agreed. He shook his head sadly.

'A tamponade that size? Not in my hands and not on my watch. That's not survivable at all. To save her, you'd have to open the chest first and find and stop the source of all the bleeding. It's a similar problem to Princess Diana's injury. No, definitely not survivable.'

Princess Diana Spencer had died as the result of injuries sustained in a high-speed car crash in the Pont de l'Alma tunnel back in 1997. She had a small tear in the low-pressure vein carrying blood to her lung. That passes very close by the spot where Helen's fatal wound had occurred and it's the devil's own job to get to it surgically. I could attest to that. It was hard enough for me to do in the mortuary, but very much more complicated when the cavity you're working in is awash with blood and you're working almost blind through a much smaller incision. The injury to the Princess was relatively small, but even with rapid access to great surgical and resuscitation facilities, she couldn't be saved.

An investigation into the Armed Offenders Squad's reaction time was subsequently conducted. Judge Ian Borrin, who was presiding, decided that they weren't slow to respond, and in fact, all of their actions were commendable and performed to the highest standards of professionalism. It was probably also some comfort to Helen's family, who had suffered all the media speculation about chances to rescue her being lost, that Judge Borrin accepted Bruce's opinion that Helen's wounds were not surgically survivable in the circumstances.

I was called to give evidence in the trial of Douglas Thompson. It was all pretty routine. I was being asked questions and was giving my answers, painfully and unnaturally slowly so that the court stenographers could keep pace. Every now and then, I was asked to stop and spell an unfamiliar word. It has to be like this, when for the purposes of open justice, court proceedings are recorded this way. But it makes delivering and hearing even straightforward testimony a wearying ordeal. For court officers, judges and juries, it must be like suffering Parkinsonism.

Then a question from Saul Holt, the quick-witted, silver-tongued Crown prosecutor, took me by surprise.

'Doctor, is it true that you were familiar with gunshot wounds in Africa?'

I agreed, eyeing Saul warily. What was he up to?

'Were most, if not all, of those injuries, sustained in the Rhodesian civil war?'

'Yes, that is correct.'

'So you're familiar with the effects of gunshot injury?'

Of course I was.

'Would you say you've had experience of hundreds of such wounds?'

'Yes. In both the living and the dead.'

'Thank you. No further questions.'

And that was it. I was left wondering what the hell it was all about. I only learned years later when Saul was off to Australia to live. At a farewell function, I asked him about it.

'Oh, that,' he said. 'That was a great moment for me.'

'Why?'

Witnesses can't hear any evidence that's led before they're called to give theirs, so I had no idea what had happened before me. Apparently, the court had heard evidence about the range at which it was likely the rifle had been fired, and of course, the defence had done their job and worked hard to create doubt in the minds of the jury members.

'You gave your opinion and it was easy to follow the reasoning,' Saul explained. 'So then I thought I'd seal the deal by pointing out that you'd seen quite a few gunshot wounds before. The jury were greatly impressed with that and I reckon they decided you must be right.'

Of course, warfare injuries with high-velocity assault rifles are not quite the same as those inflicted in a murder committed using a .22 rifle: the range at which a soldier has been shot is pretty irrelevant, to start with. Nonetheless, I am still confident that my interpretation was the right one, and indicated a particularly cold-blooded element to the murders. The jury agreed. Douglas Thompson was sentenced to life imprisonment with a 12-year minimum non-parole term. He was released after 13. We like to think that once you've done your time, that's that, but often it doesn't work out that way. Redemption is a hard road and New Zealand is a small country where everyone is pretty much aware of who the other joker is and what he's done. Thompson was prohibited from living in the Manawatu or Rangitikei districts, where Helen's family were. No-one wants to bump into their mother's killer, no matter how many years have passed.

But there was a hiccup. He settled in Panama Village, a retirement home in Masterton, where, coincidentally, a friend of Helen's daughter was also living. Helen's daughter predictably bumped into Thompson when she was visiting there. It was a horrible shock for her and her friend, although not one that could have been foreseen. I guess you have to live somewhere when you are released, but provincial New Zealand is a small place.

Paul Allen. 16 December 2001. Requiescat in pace.
Helen Johns. 16 December 2001. Requiescat in pace.

CHAPTER 7

The Cancer Wakes

'What can I do to help you?'

The woman in the bed in the day ward at Palmerston North Hospital smiled at me wearily. A bag of blood dripped slowly into the veins of her arm. Her eyes were unnaturally large and bright but serene, although I could see that her face was drawn, as those of terminal patients often are.

'I would like my story to be told. I would like people to know me when I have died and am gone. And you can do an autopsy on me, if you like. See what's going on, if you think it might be useful.'

It's the job of pathologists to find the answers to which death and disease are the questions. But it's not often that we set out on that search at the explicit behest of the patient. It is an honour to be given that gift. I didn't reply right away. I went away and thought it through carefully, and asked Elayne what she thought. Then I returned to Christine Chambers' hospital ward and gave her my answer.

'Christine, I'm honoured to be offered the opportunity to autopsy you. But I can't accept. At the end, you'll need to be with your family. They'll have their own farewells to make and we mustn't interfere with that. But do you know "autopsy" means "to see for myself"? Well, we *have* seen you for ourselves. We know you as well as we're ever going to get to know you. I'll tell your story. It won't be buried away.'

* * *

I had first met Christine in my lab. There was a piece of her on the platform of my microscope. Not long before, it had been brought in by Richard Coutts, a charismatic general surgeon and the son of and worthy successor to John Coutts. It was a biopsy, and after it had been prepared — thinly sliced, stained with dye to highlight salient features and mounted on a glass slide — I bent to the eyepiece of the microscope as Richard jiggled expectantly from foot to foot behind me.

'What's the verdict?' he chirped. 'Is it TB?'

It was typical of Richard to pursue his patients' results hot off the press. He was often there shortly after the samples had arrived from the theatre where he had extracted them by biopsy, sometimes even before we could decide what we were seeing.

I straightened up.

'It's all necrotic, I'm afraid. It could be lymphoma, but it's just not good enough for a diagnosis.'

'Necrotic' means the tissue is dead and has broken down to an unrecognisable mush.

'Bugger!' he said cheerfully. 'That's done it. You know this is going to end up a surgical disaster?'

'Why? Just biopsy us a whole node and not one that's dead and we'll get you the diagnosis.'

He shook his head.

'I'll have to open her up. The nodes are all plastered onto large blood vessels and I'll tear those open for sure when I grub them out. She'll have a catastrophic haemorrhage and I can't fix that through a laparoscope.' A laparoscope is a flexible tube equipped with a light, camera and a variety of grabbing and cutting instruments that have made it possible to perform all kinds of internal surgeries without making the inches-long incision that conventional surgery usually requires. 'She'll be lucky if I don't cause a major vascular injury as well. By the way, did you know her brother died at the same age from an intra-abdominal lymphoma?'

That was interesting. Could there be a link? I couldn't immediately think of one.

'Lymphoma's not usually thought to be one of those cancers that are inherited, though,' I replied.

'The stakes are pretty high here, then. Ah well. I'd better get on with it.'

Richard wasn't a surgeon who would shy away from risks, not when his patients' lives were hanging in the balance. He would go to the end of the road, no matter how difficult. He explained it all to Christine.

'It's horribly risky but I'll give it a go through the laparoscope. You realise that you might have a catastrophic bleed that I can't control?'

Christine nodded.

'And even if I can staunch it, you might go into multi-organ failure. That would be fatal.'

It was, as Richard related it, a sombre discussion. But Christine was a resolute woman and nothing would deter her. She was just going to do this.

Not long afterwards, Richard came bouncing ecstatically into the lab wearing his surgical scrubs. Above his head, he waved a transparent plastic biohazard bag in which there was a specimen pot.

'Paths!' he boomed. 'Look what I've got for you! A real treat for the registrars!' He whirled the bag around. I could see a bloodied nubbin of tissue bouncing about within the pot. 'Still warm! I've kept it fresh so you can do markers and send it for TB culture!'

The infection control inspectors would have conniptions. But this was typical Richard. On his operating days, we were used to him bursting in, triumphantly holding aloft a plastic bag filled with a fresh, gory pancreas or spleen or stomach. He would slap whatever it was wetly onto our desks like some Aztec priest's propitiatory sacrifice.

As usual, we all — pathologists and registrars — looked up from our microscopes to hear Richard's story.

'I thought I'd have a look down the laparoscope and see if there was a node I could winkle out. As today is Christine's birthday, I figured it was worth a go to give her a present rather than open her up.'

Richard's eyes were sparkling with happiness. It was catching, and I couldn't help but feel happy, too.

'I've got you a good one, all right! Big and juicy! But I reckon I was within a cell or two of carving a hole in her internal iliac vein! I just managed to snaffle it off the vein without bursting it.'

I took the pottle containing the node and squinted up at it.

'Doesn't look like TB to me.'

We always hope for TB rather than lymphoma in our patients. We can invariably cure tuberculosis, but lymphoma is much, much harder, especially for the patient.

'Well, you'd better get the diagnosis with that node,' Richard said. 'I'm not going back in there. I reckon I've used up all my luck today.'

He was right. It *was* a great node, big and juicy. It should have been fine. But it was dead, completely necrotic, too. And to add humility to our hubris, a complication flared up. Christine developed an abscess beside her belly button where Richard had punctured a hole through which to pass his laparoscope. Richard found her down in the Emergency Department with the red and angry tuberous swelling at the port site of her belly button. I later heard of the conversation he'd had with Christine's GP.

'I offered her either a general anaesthetic and drainage, waiting days and days for the hospital to organise it. Or I said I could just hold her down in the clinic like in the American Civil War and lash it open without anaesthesia. She opted for the latter. This is an indicator of her resilient personality. Despite carving out most of the largest node she has, the pathologists are prevaricating on the exact nature of her lymphoma. I have already put her at considerable risk during this procedure and I don't think there's any other suitable lesion I can biopsy.'

I discussed Christine's case with Elayne. Elayne is a haematologist and, by now, Christine was her patient. 'This node was totally necrotic, too. It must be her immune system that's knocking them off. Whatever is in there, her body is just killing it off faster than we can biopsy it. I can tell you one thing for sure, though, it's definitely not tuberculosis.'

'It sounds like a large B-cell lymphoma to me,' said Elayne. 'I've seen them do this before.'

'Would you ever just treat it on spec?'

What I meant by this was treating for the suspected disease without a formal diagnosis. We used to call it a 'trial of treatment' back in Africa, where we had few diagnostic tools to help us. I knew the answer before I asked the question, of course. This wasn't Africa, after all.

'I'd like to,' Elayne said, shaking her head. 'But I've discussed this with all the haematologists and they all say definitely not. The treatment is so toxic it may kill her. We just can't do it without the evidence to back us up.'

And so the hunt went on for that elusive evidence. More needles were pushed deep into Christine's abdomen; more cores were bored out of her lymph nodes. Trouble was, all were necrotic. The answer remained maddeningly out of reach.

Then, one evening, a little light appeared on the horizon. Elayne and I were bathed in the aroma of our dinner cooking, chatting and catching up on the news of one another's day.

'Christine is better!' she exclaimed. 'She came to see me today and she says it's gone!'

I frowned sceptically.

'How can it be gone? Nodes don't just *go*. *Where's* it gone?' Pathologists see too much of the hard end of life and death and disease to believe in such improbably happy endings.

'We were about to start treatment for lymphoma, out of desperation, really. Now Christine has come in and says she suddenly realised she feels fine. All her symptoms have gone and she feels normal again. I didn't believe her, of course, so I did a CAT scan to check. She's right! The nodes have gone. Shrunken away to nothing.'

Elayne was looking thoughtful, as though she could hardly believe it herself. But she had seen the evidence with her own eyes. She was thinking through the possible explanations.

'You know, she travels regularly to Thailand. Her shop sells all sorts of clothes. She sources a lot from Thailand, so she travels over there every year. Couldn't this all be a viral illness of some sort? Like that weird Kikuchi lymphadenitis they get in the East? Doesn't that mimic lymphoma?'

It was a good thought. There are many viruses that produce illnesses that can look like lymphoma.

'It doesn't look like Kikuchi's to us,' I replied. 'Besides, I thought you'd already looked for infectious mononucleosis and herpes and all those viruses?'

'Yes, we have and everything is negative,' Elayne said. 'But what if it's some exotic virus that you only get in Thailand? One we don't test for or know about. Like that dengue fever you got from mosquitoes in Fiji?'

'That's not exotic. At least, not in Fiji. It's like the common cold there. Was she bitten by any insects in Thailand?'

'Not that we know of.' Elayne shrugged. 'We'll just have to wait and see. There's nothing else to be done at the moment. But it is very good news.'

It *was* very good news. Richard Coutts was overjoyed when I passed it on.

'That's great! So what caused it in the end?'

'Who knows? Maybe some virus, some Thai insect bite. But whatever it was, it seems to have gone.'

None of us know the future, do we?

* * *

The Cancer Wakes

Christine told me all about her upbringing when I finally got to meet her in person. She grew up at the eastern end of the Port Hills above Christchurch. The rolling hills are as green as any in New Zealand and fertile, too. When you stand upon Scarborough Hill, you overlook the azure ocean that reaches from the distant horizon to where, close beneath you, lines of breaking surf scallop its edges as they surge into the bay and onto the wide, grey expanse of Sumner Beach.

Christine and her brother had an idyllic childhood roaming their slice of paradise in the valley above the beach. It was the 1960s. Their grandfather was a market gardener, and they were free to play amongst the fields of vegetables, playing hide-and-go-seek in the orchards and chasey up and down the lanes between the frames bearing the berry canes. Not only did they have a millionaire's view, but their food was as good as anyone could wish for, too. It was all proudly grown, tended and harvested by their own family.

I nodded at that.

'All of our food came off the farm, too. Our vegetables and our fruit. My mother made all of our jams and even our tomato sauce. We always had plenty to eat. And we grew up strong and healthy. I guess most Kiwi kids were the same.'

Christine told me how it was she discovered her illness.

'I was feeling really unwell with a bit of stomach pain, so I went to my GP. He couldn't find anything much so he sent me off, saying it would all just get better.'

I nodded at that one, too. The story of a doctor missing the first symptom is as old as medicine itself. I had heard it often enough and it usually ended the same, too. The difficulty facing a GP when presented with a bunch of non-specific symptoms such as Christine's is how to winnow out those very few with a critical pathology from the thousands who will recover with nothing diagnosed. It was the prospect of facing that insoluble dilemma day in, day out that convinced me I should become a pathologist in the first place.

'Anyway, it didn't get better. So I went back and was sent for an ultrasound.'

'I suppose he was thinking of gallstones?' I guessed.

Christine was in her fifties and on the plump side. She unashamedly told me she loves food, and is particularly fond of chocolate almonds — but then, who isn't? She had never done anything so ridiculous as going on a diet or trying to lose weight. At medical school, they had told us that the perfect profile for gallstones was 'female, fat, fertile and fifty'.

Christine shook her head.

'He was wondering about woman's problems. Yes, that's what he actually said! But there wasn't anything to be found, really. They did eventually look for gallstones, but all they found was a big lymph gland, deep in the back of my stomach. "Keep an eye on that gland." That was the advice I was given! How can you keep an eye on something in the back of your abdomen?'

Christine laughed, a laugh so cheerful and full of life that I couldn't help but laugh with her.

'Then we came to live in Foxton Beach and I found a new GP in Otaki. He could see something was wrong and arranged for a CAT scan. And there it was. There were lots of big lymph glands everywhere and even growing into my bladder. A needle was stuck into one of them and a biopsy taken.'

That lump of tissue was my first meeting with Christine. I had come to know her better and in person close to a year on from the moment where I first failed to give her a definitive diagnosis from that biopsy of her necrotic lymph node. Because a year on, the brilliant news that Elayne had shared with me about Christine's spontaneous cure had proved to be a false dawn.

The illness was back with a vengeance. Yet another needle had been plunged deeply through her skin, through the subcutaneous fat and into her abdominal cavity. More cores of tissue had been cut from the lymph nodes lying alongside the aorta. At last, we had been presented with an intact sample, with no necrosis. I had gazed intently down my microscope, trimmed wheels to bring it into focus — and my heart had sunk. The sunlight had suddenly seemed dimmer than before. There was no longer any doubt. A diffuse large B-cell lymphoma was present and permeating the tissues.

With the culprit now clearly defined, Elayne and the rest of the haematologists were given the call to arms and they plunged in with their heaviest artillery. They would need all of this and more to pull Christine back. You may wonder what more there might be than the full arsenal of chemotherapeutic drugs. Well, there is one thing. There is always that undefinable something, a matter of luck, fate, chance or whatever you want to call it, that causes some treatments to be effective where others, in apparently identical cases, are not. Christine had already kept this beast at bay once, fighting it all but out of existence with her own, unaided immune system. There was reason to hope that her body and the chemo would work together to defeat it.

By the time I met her, however, that hope had faded. The battle had been fiercely fought. One by one, every useful cancer drug we had was hurled at the disease. Sometimes, one or another of them seemed to be working. Then, for no apparent reason, it wouldn't be working any more. It was like a game of Snakes and Ladders, with ever fewer ladders and more and more snakes.

'I am just so thankful my doctors have never stopped and have never given up these last two years,' Christine said to me.

She wasn't what I'd expected, but perhaps that was because I didn't really know what to expect. Pathologists really have little idea of living patients. Before we met, Christine had only been a biopsy to me, an intellectual exercise, one of thousands we diagnose every day, every week and every month. In the flesh, Christine was beautifully and colourfully dressed. Of course she was. As a fashionista, a designer and purveyor of high-end women's apparel, how could she be otherwise?

'How are you feeling now?' I asked.

'Very well, really,' she replied. 'I know I haven't long. I know that I'm dying. I just take every day, one day at a time.'

'Believe me, we all should do that. As a pathologist, I can tell you that life is always full of the unexpected. Death is one of those unexpected things. As we talk here, now, there are the living walking amongst us today, on Tuesday, who don't know that on Thursday morning, they will be lying cold in my mortuary awaiting their autopsy. Their weekend plans are all in vain. This will be a bad week for them. In fact, it will be the worst week of their entire lives.'

Christine laughed again.

'I needed to go back to Thailand to renew this year's orders, but Elayne wouldn't let me. She says the lymphoma is too far advanced. My kidneys are blocked with lymphoma and I might die at any moment. The chances of me dying on the way are too high to risk. Or I could end up ill over there with no medical help and no insurance.'

'That's a pretty definite prognosis,' I said, wondering what else I could say. This was not the sort of conversation I'm accustomed to. 'But you've had a hell of an immune reaction to the cancer already with all those necrotic nodes. Who can tell? Maybe it'll happen again?'

It was the best I could think of.

'I'll have to hurry, then. Elayne has promised to keep me going until my birthday on the 31st of May. And my family are on holiday in Bali until then. I've got to wait until they come home before I shuffle off.'

That was only three weeks hence: exactly two years since Richard's first heart-stopping biopsy, and one year since I first saw the enemy in sharp focus through my microscope. Now I really didn't know what to say. Christine laughed yet again.

'I decided I didn't want a big funeral. I am not that sort of person at all. Life is there to be lived. So I decided to have a wedding instead.'

'A wedding? Whose?'

'Why, mine, of course! My grandchildren were so sad when I told them I was dying, but you should have seen the excitement on my granddaughter's face when I told her about the wedding. You see, Blue and I had never got married, even after 37 years. It just seemed like a good time.'

'You really are a "glass half-full" person, aren't you?'

'I am more than that,' she beamed. 'I think I've got a full set of glasses and they're all beautiful! Instead of a funeral, we had the wedding. It was supposed to be on Foxton Beach but there were so many people coming that we had to have it in

Foxton Beach School Hall. It was wonderful! There were 75 people there and it was everything I could have wished for.'

'And now? Is there anything else you need to do?'

'Oh yes. I went to the undertaker to arrange my funeral. I call it my "dispatch shopping".'

That laugh again.

'That's pretty different.' I grinned. 'How did the undertaker react? Was he embarrassed?'

'A little, at first, but he was quite professional, really. I chose my coffin.' Christine nodded proudly. 'It was an easy choice. I only wanted the cheap one. After all, it's only going to be burned.'

We both became a little pensive. We're not very good at talking about death, especially our own. Christine was better at talking about it than most, but even she was haunted by some of the unknowns.

'Why did this happen to me?' she asked quietly. 'It was those chemicals, wasn't it? It must have been. My brother died at only 58 with exactly the same cancer as mine and in the same place. All my family who lived there have died young from cancer.'

Talking about her childhood, Christine had told me about the chemical sprays her grandfather had used in his gardens and orchards.

'I used to play alongside while my grandfather worked when I was younger. But as I got older, I helped out whenever I could. I didn't really have to do too much, but I was always there. Granddad always wore shorts and no shirt and he was baked brown by the sun. The spray was a mist that went everywhere. My grandfather used to come in drenched in it after a day's work.'

'I guess there was no protection in those days?' I asked. 'Like masks, for instance?'

'No.' Christine shook her head and smiled at me. 'No, there was nothing like that. I played in and out of the spray, too. No-one thought it strange and no-one stopped me. I can still remember the smell and taste of it quite vividly, after 50 years.'

I nodded. My sister and her husband had farmed in the wilds of Zambia and, in later years, on the sloping sides of the Franschhoek mountains of the Western Cape. I knew that insecticides were common and critical for crop survival back in those days. The dangers of DDT, which had been the most widely used pesticide in the earlier part of the twentieth century, were well known by then, and 'safe' alternatives had been brought to the market. Like Christine's grandfather, my brother-in-law used dieldrin, which was one of these alternatives. I remember the smell of it, too: it used to make me feel good, imagining it killing all those pests and leaving our wholesome food for us to gather to sell and eat. Dieldrin was used worldwide during the 1950s and right up to the late 1970s. It doesn't break down easily and persists in the food chain, becoming ever more concentrated as you eat sources contaminated with it. And it causes cancer. Dieldrin and other organochloride pesticides were finally completely banned in New Zealand only in 1995. God only knows what it did to us all in the meantime.

It may well have been the chemicals that started the time bomb ticking in Christine's lymphatic system. There may have been something else, too, like some sort of inherited, genetic susceptibility that she shared with her brother. But if I had to place a bet, it would be dollars to doughnuts that it was the chemicals.

Medicine is just a science, in the end, and with the newspapers so full of the amazing successes and breakthroughs made in medicine, people are often surprised at what we can't do. Sometimes, no matter how hard we try, we just cannot get a diagnosis. We may only find the cause of death at autopsy, too late to be of any help to the patient. It's even harder to understand when we do have a diagnosis but the treatment fails abjectly. At this stage of our knowledge, we just don't know why, but it is heartbreaking for us all.

I couldn't give Christine an answer to her question. We were pretty sure we knew the what, where and how of her disease: hers was an enemy that we know of old. But we do not know the why of how it came or why the treatment failed in her case. That puzzle is in the hands of the diligent medical researchers in their sophisticated laboratories.

Christine Chambers. 20 June 2019. Requiescat in pace.

Death closes all: but something ere the end
Some work of noble note, may yet be done.
—Alfred, Lord Tennyson, 'Ulysses' (1842)

* * *

'I understand. I'll let the patient know and call you back if she's ready to have another go.'

I had half-woken as I heard the phone ring, and as I heard Elayne speak those words, I came fully awake. I knew from long experience that my efforts to go back to sleep would be futile: a bed shared by a pathologist and a haematologist is a recipe for sleep disturbance.

The only consolation was that the call wasn't for me. I pulled the covers over my head to hide from the light that I knew was about to flood the room. I heard Elayne sigh heavily, and the bed shifted as she sat up, dialled a number and began talking.

'Hello, Jackie. I've got your results and I'm afraid the harvest failed. You'll need to go right now up to Ward 25 to get another booster injection and come back first thing tomorrow and we'll try again.'

There was a pause. Then the person on the other end spoke. Despite my hood of blankets, I could clearly hear every word.

'Oh no! What happened?'

'We were trying to harvest your bone marrow stem cells from your blood. The injections to wake them up and get them into your blood haven't done the trick. We just didn't get enough for us to go ahead with your treatment.'

'Does this mean you can't treat me now?'

My duvet couldn't dull the edge of anguish.

'No, there are other things we can do. But first we'll try again tonight to push your cell levels up and see if we can improve the harvest to a workable level in the morning.'

This was a conversation I had heard a dozen times before. I wasn't going to get back to sleep just like that, so I decided to settle for the hour and a half I'd had.

'What's this harvest for?' I asked.

'It's Jackie. You know her. Jacqueline. She's one of the senior clerical staff down near the surgeons' offices. You've seen her bone marrow before.'

'I remember. Myeloma. You want to do a bone marrow transplant?'

'The painkillers haven't really touched it.' Elayne sounded concerned. 'I don't think this is going to end well. She really needs that transplant.'

I was sorry to hear this. Of course I knew Jackie, and not just from her bone marrow slides. We often met at the same door coming into work just after seven each morning. She was often to be seen busily pushing a trolley with piles of patient files around the corridors.

Bone marrow transplants are performed in cases where the body's capacity for manufacturing blood cells has been destroyed. These can be wiped out by a variety of diseases — of these, leukaemia is the most widely known, and feared — but it can also be caused by the chemotherapy used as a treatment for cancers. The idea that you could replace diseased bone marrow with healthy tissue is an old one, but it wasn't until 1956 that it was first performed successfully, using marrow from one of a pair of identical twins to treat the other. They've come a long way since Elayne and I had first been involved in them in the 1980s in Cape Town. Back then, all our transplants were from a matched donor to the patient, just as organ transplants — such as kidney and heart and liver — still are today. Elayne's team did them. It was a horrible procedure, and the results were pretty appalling, too. Marrow was sucked out through large, wide-bore needles plunged repeatedly into the donor's hip bones. Bags of sieved and separated bloody marrow were run hopefully into the patient's veins. Battle was then joined. The body's immediate reaction was to reject this massive assault by foreign bodies: immunosuppressive drugs were administered to damp this response down. Sometimes they worked. Often they didn't, and then I did the autopsies on their waxen, wasted bodies, the skin peeling off from rejection and their organs stuffed with a zoo of bacteria, viruses and moulds of creeping fungi. They were horrible. It seemed to me a case of heads you lose from rejection, tails you lose from infection. And even if the battle against infection and rejection was won, the original leukaemia could return and the war could be lost anyway.

Nowadays, injections are administered that overstimulate the production of so-called 'stem cells' — the 'Adam and Eve cells' of the body, that can turn into the other kinds of cells that comprise our various, specialised tissues. The excess stem cells are gently siphoned from the patient's blood. The patient is then given a dose of a toxic anti-cancer drug that destroys their cancerous bone marrow, leaving their bones not only clean of any hidden cancer, but also with no surviving normal blood-making cells. This would be lethal under normal circumstances. But the harvested stem cells are run back into their bloodstream, and just like the cavalry, they charge to the rescue, piling into the void and recolonising the empty marrow mesh. It's a lifesaving miracle.

Jackie had myeloma, an aggressive blood cancer. It was treatable, but only if her body could be chemically persuaded to produce enough stem cells to rescue her from the lethal dose of chemotherapy it would need. So far, it had not.

'How did it actually start?' I asked Jackie.

'I thought I'd pulled a muscle in my back. I went to a physio and had massages, but it didn't help at all.'

Jackie is a calm person and, I sensed, a stoical and strong woman. I imagined her capacity to suffer pain would be high, probably even exceptionally high.

'I saw so many GPs. Each time I went, it was someone different. I'm not a complainer but they didn't seem to realise how bad I was. I couldn't sit up straight. I used to go tramping up the Otaki Forks, but I just couldn't carry my pack any more. It got so bad that even when my trolley bumped into the gap between the door and the floor in the hospital lift, the jolt tore down into my back and the pain was just overwhelming. I wasn't giving up coming to work, so in my lunch hours I used to go and lie on my back in the Garden of Tranquillity to try to ease it.'

I knew the place. The Garden of Tranquillity is a charming courtyard garden next to the chapel and opposite the Mental Health Unit. It's a quiet place to meditate, perhaps, but all the peace and quiet and meditation in the world won't beat the pain from a hidden cancer.

'Eventually, a few days before Christmas, I was sent for an X-ray of my back. The bones of my spine had collapsed. That was the cause of my pain, they said. But no-one looked at it until much later, because Christmas came on in between. I just carried on.'

'The X-ray gave them the diagnosis, I suppose?'

'No, they thought that it was just osteoporosis. That my bones were thinning but this was to be expected in a woman of my age. I just couldn't believe it! I had exercised and kept fit all my life. How could my bones just be broken like that?'

'So how did you find out?'

'It was six months later. My GP did a blood test and discovered I was in kidney failure. Then everything just happened. I was rushed up to the hospital and saw the renal doctors and then soon after that I ended up with Elayne in Haematology. It was hard to believe.'

The Cancer Wakes

Her first meeting with my wife was not the nicest, as you can imagine.

'Jackie, the news is not great,' Elayne said. Jackie and her partner, Geoff, were sitting anxiously in her clinic. 'You've got a cancer of your blood. I am pretty sure this is a myeloma, which is a cancer of some of the lymphocytes in your blood. The cancer has spread to your spine, which is why your vertebrae have collapsed. It's also all through your marrow, so you're anaemic. And it has involved your kidney, too, which is why you're in kidney failure. I'll need to biopsy your bone marrow so we can confirm this and it will help us learn more about what type it is and how we may treat it.'

Jackie and Geoff were dumbfounded, although I'll bet Jackie knew something was up. People usually do.

The confirmation came quick and fast after all those months of waiting, of uncertainty.

'Look at this.' Elayne handed me a microscope slide. I looked down. There was a stained, tubular core of tissue on the glass — a bone marrow trephine, a biopsy taken with a large-bore needle from the back of her hip bone. 'What do you think?'

The bone marrow was stuffed full of blue cells. Blue is bad, in my business. We apply dyes to tissue samples that highlight diseased cells which show up blue under visible light. I looked under the highest power and the cells looked up at me, each dressed in a coat of imperial purple cytoplasm, with faces like a clock and a subtle toothy smile.

'Plasma cells? Myeloma?' Nothing smiley about those cells. They were deadly killers at large. Their nuclei looked like clock faces, marking time that was running out for the patient.

Elayne nodded. 'More than 90 per cent are malignant cells. The normal marrow is wiped out. She's got a free kappa chain level of fourteen thousand, too.'

Free kappa chains. 'Free' is a feel-good word in most contexts, but there was nothing to feel good about with kappa chains. Kappa chains are twists of protein made by malignant plasma cells and they plug up the kidneys, so badly that it soon becomes irreversible. The only hope is aggressive treatment. Myeloma is relentless, and the treatment has to be too. It's like a terrible game of double or quits.

Jackie entered the whirl of the cancer treatment service. 'It all happened too fast for me to follow easily and I am not really medical. I just had to trust my doctors and they were great. Elayne gave me a lot of confidence.'

Healing radiation was directed at her collapsed spine. Drugs were poured into her bloodstream — a mixed blessing, because the drugs destroy the healthy cells even as they cure the diseased body. Cancer therapy is always a tightrope balance between doing good and harm.

'It was the pain that I remember,' said Jackie. 'It was exquisite, worse than anything I could imagine.'

Exquisite pain. That is what many who have suffered myeloma remember with clarity. The voracious, malignant cells break and breach the scaffold of your bones one minute lamella at a time. It is like having your bones fractured slowly over days and weeks. The only pain that comes close is that intense pain you get deep in the bones of your legs when you unwisely venture into the icy winter sea or into a glacial river. It is a pain that is so visceral it makes you vomit. And as Jackie could attest, the treatment can be as bad as the symptom.

'The pain relief was dreadful. The morphine, the methadone, the gabapentin, the green skin patches — they just made me hallucinate and shiver and I felt even worse than before.'

I remembered.

'Yes, the radiation oncologists said that you were so bad they couldn't even have a meaningful discussion with you. They were worried your shaking was because you had septicaemia. They had no choice but to hold back until you'd made some progress and got your pain and your kidney failure under control. It may have been pain from the nerves trapped beneath your fallen spine but there's no doubt it was creeping death you were feeling in your bones.'

Things were really bleak by this stage. The cancer was everywhere. Her marrow, her ribs, her spine, her skull and even her jaw were involved. Jackie was sent to the palliative care doctors at the hospice asking them to control her pain. It wasn't easy, but they were compassionate and persistent.

And then against the flow of expectation, against the relentless flood tide of bad news, bad signs and advanced disease, there arose a glimmer of hope. The twisted kappa chain proteins melted away from Jackie's bloodstream like an ice-cream in the noonday desert sun. From 14,000 to 300 the chains dropped, and then further to an incredible 40, all in just two months.

The pain was still there and still intense, but Jackie thought the edge might have come off it. She wasn't sure. After so long in such agony, you hope it's going, but can you dare to be sure of anything?

'The pain you still have is definitely because of pinched nerves and not advancing disease,' Elayne decided. 'It's now time to move on to the next stage. You're ready for bone marrow transplantation.'

* * *

So here we were, closing in on midnight for the second night running, and I was resigned to another disturbed night. Would Jackie do it this time? Would the stem cell harvest be fruitful?

Alas, when the call came, it was bad news. It had failed, again.

This seemed very hard on Jackie.

'Why?' I asked. 'Does this often happen?'

Elayne shook her head. 'No, it's very unusual. I just have no idea why.'

She made the call to break the sad news to Jackie.

'What happens now?' I asked, after she'd finished the call. 'How does this affect things?'

'We carry on with the next consolidation course of chemotherapy. On to thalidomide.'

Thalidomide. Now there was a name to conjure up horrors from the past! Thalidomide was freely sold over the counter in the 1950s and early 1960s to pregnant women to relieve morning sickness — even for some time after the reports of horrendous side effects began to pile up. Over ten thousand infants were born without arms or legs or both. Many had heart and eye defects. Sixty per cent of them died. The drug was soon banned, of course, and thereafter only discussed in hushed tones. Forty years on, it was found to be pretty good against myeloma and quietly reinstated into the medical mainstream.

Because of its catastrophic effects on unborn children, all myeloma patients, men and women, have to sit through and listen like teenagers to a 'no babies' lecture before they're allowed to start their thalidomide. Elayne was obliged to counsel Jackie and Geoff about the dangers of getting pregnant, and even gave them an official letter warning them against it. This provided a moment of light relief on the otherwise sombre journey: with her levels of pain, doing anything that might result in Jackie getting pregnant was most certainly off the cards!

People are often amazed at doctors' failures, but cancer is not easy. We often have to inch our way two steps forward and then one back for months at a time. Jackie developed an intensely itchy rash over her body as a reaction to the thalidomide.

'I'll stop the thalidomide,' Elayne told Jackie. 'But it's not all bad news. So far as we can tell, the myeloma has gone. The radiation has stabilised your spine, and your kidneys have now settled down and are working steadily. Because your response has been so good, I want to stop your treatment now and watch and see how you get on.'

'Will my pain go?' Jackie asked, conditioned by her recent experience not to dare to hope for even more good news.

'We can't undo the damage that's been done. That's always there, I'm afraid.'

'Will the myeloma come back? Has it gone?'

'I don't know for sure,' Elayne admitted. 'But it's certainly gone for now and I'm not expecting it back. But I will see you every few months to check.'

It did not return. We had won.

'I wanted to ask you,' Jackie said to me, years later. 'Could I have got my myeloma from a spray? I used a spray to kill the ragwort in my garden and I could smell and taste it all the time I was using it. Did that cause the myeloma, do you think?'

'What did you use? Some chemicals have been associated with myeloma.'

'I think it was called Tordon.'

I looked it up. Under the code name Agent White, it was used as a chemical defoliant during the Vietnam War. Unlike its more infamous cousin, Agent Orange (with which it shares an ingredient), it has not been shown to be toxic to humans.

'I grew up in Feilding and other places around here, where my father was a gardener by profession. He would have used chemical sprays but I don't think I was any more exposed than anyone else.'

'Who can tell now, Jackie?' I answered. 'I reckon we were all probably exposed to those chemicals more than we realised, way back then. Everyone used them. We just didn't think about it. And their long-term effects are just unknown.'

It has been nine years since I first saw Jackie's cancer cells down my microscope and today I often see her hurrying about the hospital still pushing her trolley. I feel a jolt of happiness whenever I do. It makes this job worthwhile and it's good to know that sometimes the treatment does work wonders.

And now I see with eye serene
The very pulse of the machine:
A being breathing thoughtful breath:
A traveller betwixt life and death.
—William Wordsworth, 'She was a Phantom of Delight' (1807)

CHAPTER 8

Death at the Chicken Ranch

July mornings can be icy in the Manawatu.

It was a quarter to seven on a Saturday morning and I was concentrating on not cutting myself as I carefully shaved the foam off my upper lip. My feet were bare and the winter chill had insinuated itself through the ceramic bathroom tiles. As always, I told myself that I should really have put my slippers on. I never do, as they're soft, brown sheepskin and I'm a messy shaver. I can't seem to help dropping globs of stubble-bearing lather over my feet.

The phone rang.

I left it for Elayne to answer in the kitchen. Early-morning calls are far from unusual for us, and they're invariably for Elayne. Her many haematology patients are spread across the North Island and they suffer a multitude of blood problems from clots to bleeding, from fevers to fatigue and everything in between. Provincial patients are staunch folk, and they don't let on about their problems until dawn has broken. They don't want to disturb us: six-thirty or seven seems to be the time they judge it's okay to call Elayne.

'It's for you!' Elayne called out, coming down the passage with the phone. 'It's the police.'

This was early for the police. What couldn't wait until Monday?

'Good morning, Doctor. Sorry to trouble you. We have a suspicious death we'd like you to have a look at.'

I groaned internally. There goes my Saturday, I thought. At this time on a Saturday morning, I'd put money on it being the outcome of domestic violence, the upshot of a Friday-night drinking bout.

'What's the story?' I asked.

'A male body with substantial injuries has been located at the side of the road. It looks pretty suspicious.'

'By the side of the road? Where exactly did it happen? Could it be a hit-and-run?'

'On Wylie Road. He's lying in the driveway of the chicken farm, not actually on the road. We don't think it's a hit-and-run.'

'Chicken farm?' I'd never heard of a chicken farm before, let alone around here. I was familiar with sheep, cattle, deer farms — you can't live in the Manawatu and not be — and cropping operations. But not chicken farms.

'Turk's Poultry Farm. You go across State Highway 1 towards Himatangi Beach and take the first left to Foxton on Wylie Road. It's a couple of kilometres down. You'll see all our cars. You can't miss it.'

I grabbed a quick piece of toast, though I wasn't hungry any more. I was thinking murder, and my bloodstream was full of adrenaline, a response to the anticipation of horrors yet to be faced and to the prospect of performing the meticulous kind of job I'd need to perform if my work were to be scrutinised in court. I spent some time putting my kit together and arranging for the mortuary to go on standby for a homicide. The mortuary assistant's weekend relaxation would also have to be shelved. His reaction was more one of resignation than resentment. We are responsible for such a large area that there always seems to be action of one sort or another. I've never stopped admiring my assistants' uncomplaining attitudes. It springs from a genuine empathy for our patients and their families. After all, when you work with the dead, you know there's always someone else having a much worse day than you are.

I drove along Pioneer Highway, heading south-west out of town towards the beach and the Tasman Sea receding to the distant horizon. For once, the place was easy to find, although there was a police car sealing off the Himatangi end of Wylie Road.

A policewoman came over as I wound down my window. I explained who I was, and she waved me on. 'Pass on through. You can't miss them. They're just down the road.'

I love the informality of provincial New Zealand. No papers or ID ever seemed to be needed. You are just who you say you are. It reminds you that the less-than-honest amongst us are few and generally well known to the police. This makes it easier for the police to be relaxed and informal with the public.

The first sign of the scene was a white police investigation van pulled over to the left up ahead. There were several patrol cars parked at odd angles up and down the road, like brightly coloured lollies scattered from a piñata. I recognised most of the investigating officers, familiar from so many other places. I saw my old friend Steve who was the scene of crime officer and was there in overalls and boots, smiling as usual. He handed over the disposable protection suits and caps and the tough overshoes we had to pull on awkwardly over our boots.

I had learned long ago not to wear my usual lace-up leather shoes to these gigs. Instead, I wore my warm, waterproof Crispi tramping boots. You can't tell when the scene of a crime will be wet and boggy, and it's Murphy's law that the day I don't wear my boots, the murderer will have chosen a swamp in which to dump the body.

Once I was properly kitted up and signed in, I moved on to the scene itself.

The chicken ranch wasn't what I had expected at all. It looked more like a modern factory than my idea of a farm. There was a substantial building of two, maybe three storeys surrounded, like a chicken by its chicks, with a gaggle of smaller, oblong buildings. I guessed these were where the chickens lived. All were cream-coloured and well maintained. There was a grain silo in front of the main building, and across the drive, there was a sign directing you to check in at the office before entering. The whole complex was surrounded by a high fence topped with multiple strands of what looked like electrified barbed wire. The entrance was blocked by a set of double gates, also topped with coils of barbed wire and apparently electrified. They were firmly locked.

'It looks more like a prison than a farm,' I said. 'What's with all the electricity? Chickens don't fly their coop, do they? At least I've never heard of them doing that.'

'That would be for keeping the animal activists out, not the chickens in, Doc.'

I got it. Even sleepy Foxton was a potential battleground in the war over the ethical handling of animals.

The body of a man lay on his back to the side of the gate, his arms flung out as if in supplication to heaven.

'A strange place for him to die,' I observed. 'A bit out of the way, isn't it?'

The detective nodded.

'He's unidentified at the moment. None of us here recognise him and he isn't carrying any ID. It appears he's been beaten, as he's got obvious facial injuries. But that's about all we have for the moment. No-one around here has reported any trouble last night and no-one's been reported missing as yet.'

'Who found him?'

This was a remote spot and any passing cars in the early hours would probably have whipped past the recessed drive without so much as a glance at what could easily have been a bundle of discarded rags lying there by the gate.

'Two young lads who work here called us early this morning. There's a shipment of chickens that's due on the road early today. They were due to start at five.' The policeman grinned. 'They called, but then decided to leave the body out here and just get on with loading their chickens.'

I nodded approvingly. This was provincial Kiwi pragmatism at its best. They would have decided he was pretty well dead. Better to just get on with the job they were paid to do.

The detective's grin broadened.

'Unfortunately for them, the first officer on the scene didn't like the look of them at all. They were scratched and bleeding all over. The lads reckon they were scratched from catching the chickens. They say it always happens. But they're off at the station at the moment, giving a statement.'

'Surely you don't think they could have killed him, called you and then just carried on with their work right there, like that? Hardly seems plausible!'

'Nah! Reckon they're okay. Nothing to do with them. But still, we'll ask them a few hard questions and see how their story stacks up. Just bad luck for them.'

Bad luck for them indeed. Honest workers just doing their civic duty and getting on with their jobs, and a trip down to the station to 'help the police with their inquiries' was their reward.

I was eventually allowed to make my way to the body.

The deceased was slightly built, maybe 75 kilograms, with a short, salt-and-pepper beard and long, grey-streaked hair. His hair wasn't at its best right then, matted as it was with clotted blood and dirt. I judged him to be about 60 or 65. His dress was tidy if idiosyncratic, mostly thanks to a jersey that was decorated with vertical tiger stripes interspersed with leopard spots. It was not a particularly flattering or fashionable pattern. That, at least, should make him easily identifiable, I thought.

Beneath the jersey, he was wearing a checked shirt and a T-shirt against the cold. On his lower half, he wore jeans, socks that finished below his knees and shoes. Apart from that particular jersey, his outfit was pretty much what you might wear for a Friday night out anywhere in Palmerston North. He wasn't that recognisable. His lower face was unmemorable, and the injuries to his upper face were considerable.

I could make out bone beneath deep lacerations of his forehead and one deep wound across the bridge of his nose was shaped like a star-burst. The whole of his right cheekbone was caved in, pushed down into the maxillary sinus beneath. Both eyes were black and swollen closed from bleeding. There were no defensive injuries to his hands, so he hadn't been trying to protect himself when he was killed. He wore a gold wedding ring and what looked like an expensive gold watch — although I knew enough about these things to know that it could have been one of the cheap Chinese knock-offs that had become readily available.

'It all looks like blunt trauma around the eyes and midface,' I said. 'I think this is from multiple kicks while he was down on the ground, probably unconscious. You might want to collect your suspects' boots for blood, tissue and DNA.' My thoughts turned briefly to the hapless chicken ranch lads down at the station now answering questions and making their statements. Their boots would surely prove their innocence.

'So not a hit-and-run, then?'

I shook my head.

'Wrong pattern of injury for a car versus pedestrian. Wrong place for a hit-and-run, too.' I gestured down the dead-end driveway with its locked gates. 'Unless the body was dumped here after being run over somewhere else. But this is an assault, not a traffic accident.'

There were smears of dried, brownish blood on the back of each of his hands. They were out of kilter with the rest of the pattern of injury. They puzzled me, but the day was moving on and I knew I had work to do that couldn't be delayed. In any murder investigation, the time of death is a critical ingredient. Like the salt in your food, nothing tastes right without it. We're all familiar with the testing of an alibi in criminal trials, as we come across it in nearly every crime movie and novel. Time is what determines the point at which the victim and their killer intersected.

'What do you need to do?' The detectives listened attentively as I outlined my procedures, although they'd seen all this before.

'I'm going to have to move the legs and arms a bit so I can have a feel for his degree of rigor mortis. And I'll have to roll him over slightly so I can examine his back for lividity. But more importantly, I must put a needle into his eyeball to draw some fluid for a potassium level.'

I paused. I could see they were uneasy.

'I know the eyes are within the critical injury field,' I said, 'but it's an essential test. I also need to stab a hole into the side of his belly to take his body temperature. It should be done sooner rather than later.'

'I think we'll need to get the DNA swabs done before you can do any of that,' a detective said, sounding worried.

He was right. The days when a pathologist was always the first into the scene of a murder have gone, as the result of one of the two significant changes that have overtaken murder investigation in the last 20 years or so. One is CCTV footage. The widespread introduction of CCTV covering substantial parts of our cities and towns as well as the garages scattered in between has been a game-changer. Even if the actual act of murder isn't captured on some unseen camera, the roads to and from the scene as well as the buildings and shops adjoining it are often under electronic surveillance. It becomes very difficult for a suspect to deny their proximity to a scene when their movements are captured by these little glass eyes and stored in their digital memory.

The other significant technological breakthrough has been the brilliant strides made in DNA collection and analysis. There aren't too many killings where the DNA linking murderer and victim can't be collected from some part of the murder scene by diligent work. In the absence of eyewitness evidence, a DNA match placing a suspect at the scene of the crime creates a bond with the victim that is tighter than just about any other.

I stood and watched as an ESR scientist, covered from head to foot in her protective gear, began methodically dusting the man's front, hands and face with collection swabs. Each of these was labelled and placed in airtight containers and taken into the chain of custody. This chain would remain unbroken and the specimens unsullied until the scientific testing in the ESR lab for any invisible fragments of DNA that might reveal the crucial clue.

I understood the importance of this process, but I couldn't help but feel impatient as I waited to start my own work. It was already 11 o'clock, nearly six hours after the body had been discovered.

'Over to you, Doc.'

At last. A policeman came with me to assist and take notes. First, I lifted the body's left leg up by his thigh. It was rigid with rigor mortis, the knee joint locked and unyielding. I worked my way through every joint I could reasonably reach, testing them through his clothing. They were all the same — ankles, shoulders, elbows — as well as the smaller joints of the hands. The jaw was clenched tightly closed, as though he were grimacing at his ghastly fate.

'Complete rigor mortis in all joints big and small and the jaw. In this cold, that probably means about eight to ten hours ago. That would put death between 1 and 3 a.m.'

I lifted the side of the unsightly tiger-and-leopard-themed jersey and tugged his shirt partly out of his pants. I could see that his back was a deep reddish-purple with a clearly demarcated line where the blood had drained from the higher tissue to the lower and pooled there. This was livor mortis, another handy, if imprecise, change that indicated the body's journey through the processes after death.

'There's confluent, fixed lividity. There's a bigger time range for this measure, unfortunately. The degree of change we see here comes anywhere between 10 and 20 hours. Still, it fits with late-ish Friday night as the probable target.'

I took a low-reading thermometer out of my carry bag and held it steady for a few minutes about 20 centimetres off the ground to get the air temperature. It stabilised at a surprisingly warm 16 degrees in that sunless spot. I have to say, it felt much colder to me.

I selected a scalpel and stabbed it through the muscles of the victim's flank. I pushed the thermometer through my incision until I felt it pop into the abdominal cavity. The temperature column crept up and stabilised on its level.

'Twenty-five point five degrees,' I called out, and the constable dutifully wrote it down.

'What's that mean?' he asked.

'I don't know, yet,' I replied. 'I have to take it away and do a calculation to get a time range. You see, the time it takes for his body temperature to drop depends on the outside temperature, his weight, clothing, wind and all sorts of things. I feed them all into an equation and get the best range. It's not brilliant, but it's as good a guess as any and better than most.'

I pulled my bag towards me and extracted a syringe, a needle and a blood specimen tube. Kneeling by his side, I eased the needle through the gap in the purplish, bruised flesh around his left eye and inserted it into the eyeball. I was worried that he might have bled into the eyeball during the attack and it would therefore be useless for my purposes, but to my relief, clear eyeball fluid flowed thickly into the barrel of the syringe. It was soon safely sealed within a test tube. The sodium and potassium levels in that viscous fluid, fed into a complicated equation, would also help fix his time of death.

With that, I was done — for now. The police still had an immense task ahead of them, minutely searching the scene for clues, documenting everything and making sure they missed nothing significant. They also had to try to determine just who in hell this man was, and what he had been doing in the Manawatu.

'We'll probably uplift the body by late afternoon, Doc. When do you want to do the autopsy?'

I knew there wasn't any great hurry, as the autopsy wouldn't add much to what we'd already seen.

'Not tonight. But I'll head in later today when he arrives at the mortuary and do a quick re-examination to confirm what I have already seen. I'll also needle his other eyeball to get a second potassium level for my time fix.'

I saw the officer wince as I said that. This often happens. There's just something about sticking a needle into an eyeball that makes your blood run cold, isn't there?

At six o'clock that Saturday night, I collected the second syringe of vitreous humour from his swollen right eye.

We call this fluid a 'humour', but there's nothing funny about it. The vitreous humour is a semi-solid fluid that keeps the eyeball pumped up as a tense orb. 'Humour' is just the ancient word for the bodily fluids, the balance amongst which was once thought to determine your character, your moods and your state of health. The odd name is still used as a sort of weird anachronism, I suppose, rather like the British House of Lords.

I climbed the three flights of stairs from the subterranean mortuary to the brightly lit lab and delivered the humour sample to the scientists. They fed it along the rails into a big biochemistry analyser, alongside the bloods and fluids of living patients who were waiting for their results down in the Emergency Department, the wards and the ICU.

Soon enough, I had a reading for the potassium and sodium levels in the sample. I went through to my office and consulted the tables to work out a time of death. This makes me sound a bit like an ancient soothsayer sitting by a roaring fire and consulting my almanac to make sense of the past and predict the future. In a strange sort of way, this isn't far from the truth. Although there's some science behind our methods for calculating the time of death, none of them are very robust, taken in isolation. We persist in trying to do it, probably because we'd be accused of incompetence by defence lawyers if we didn't — although the same lawyers are pretty quick to point out the irredeemable flaws and the margins of error of the methods we use when we do. We can't really win.

In the end, whatever numbers come out are the only numbers we have. The numbers thrown up by different methods can be contradictory, but thanks to the equations and tables that we have, there is more consistency in the range these days than there used to be. In the case of the unknown assault victim from the chicken farm, they all more or less aligned. The algor mortis, or temperature of the body, indicated 10.15 p.m. on Friday night, give or take a couple of hours. The eyeball potassium and sodium gave a range from 10.45 p.m. to 2.30 a.m. the same night. Close enough. Late Friday night or early Saturday morning was my best estimate. I called the result through to the CIB. I learned that, as yet, there was no identification on the body.

* * *

His identity was no clearer when, early Sunday morning, we prepared to perform the autopsy. We undressed him carefully layer by layer, searching for any evidence and photographing the body as each item was removed. It was slow and tedious, but it did give me the opportunity to examine the entire surface of his body meticulously. There was nothing new to add to what I'd already discovered by the side of the chicken ranch driveway — until I came to pull his denims down.

Pat and I were standing at the foot of the gurney, tugging at a trouser leg each. They were a slim fit so it was quite hard work. It always surprises me how difficult undressing the dead is. It's as though they're trying to preserve their modesty as long as possible. Of course, they can't help you much, and somehow their rigidity seems to make their clothing cling. The denims eventually came off in a rush. I had removed a handkerchief, lightly stained with dried blood, from the pocket, and was bundling them up to bag them to go to the ESR for blood and other testing when I felt something solid. I knew exactly what it was, right away.

I dug into his right back pocket and pulled out his wallet. The incredulous looks on the attendant police officers' faces were priceless.

The wallet was emblazoned with a skull and crossbones.

'Be careful what you wish for,' I said to the body, in the presence of this emblem of death. I opened it. It was stuffed with dozens of cards — loyalty cards for tobacconists, business cards for family and criminal lawyers and, best of all, his driver's licence, complete with photograph.

'No ID, hey?' I smiled at the police. That's what they had told me the previous day at the roadside. I guessed that somebody was going to get a bollocking for this, but to be fair, the wallet was firmly tucked away and the victim was lying on top of it. These days, you're not allowed to move or interfere with the body. Still, it wasn't often I got to get one up on the CIB and see them so discomfited.

'Glen Ronald Stinson,' I read out. Despite his horrific injuries, the photograph was clearly that of the dead man. The police officers looked at each other and shrugged. The name clearly didn't mean anything to them. One of them left the mortuary to make a phone call.

He was back in less than five minutes.

'Glen Ronald Stinson. Convicted paedophile. Currently out on bail on three charges of indecent assault and one of the attempted rape of a girl under the age of 12.'

I looked up from my work. So did everyone. We stared at the officer and then at each other.

A paedophile. Currently active, too, by the sounds of it.

That certainly changed the dynamics quite a bit. You could see that, for the police, it opened a whole different world of possibilities. There would be the parents of his victims to consider, for a start. What might I do, what might any of us do, if it was one of our own precious children who had been involved? Oh, look, we'd say, as we sipped our wine. We wouldn't resort to murder. We're civilised people. Or would we? Pray we're never in a position to find out.

I concentrated on the task at hand. His body was now naked on the table. I searched up and down the hands and forearms.

'There are no defensive injuries. So he didn't try to fend off the attack at all. If he had, there would have been cuts and bruises to his hands and along the ulnar borders of his forearms.' I held my arm up in front of my face in a protective posture. 'You see? You'd have to take any blow on the outer border of your forearm first. And there's nothing here at all to show that is what happened.'

'What about the blood smears on the back of his hands?'

I had first pointed those out at the scene as very odd and out of context. But now, since finding the bloodstained handkerchief in his pocket, I had a theory. My stellar teacher of forensic medicine, Kevin Lee, always told us to look at the evidence and imagine how it could possibly have come to be there, in the form that you had in front of you.

'I think these stains on the back of his hands pre-date the murder, possibly even by some hours. I think there was an argument of some sort earlier on and it came to blows. Stinson was punched on the nose. He didn't fight back, because there are no other fight-type injuries, which would be very different from those which killed him. No. I visualise him responding passively to this blow and standing there wiping the dribble of blood from his nose, first with the back of his right hand and then, shortly after, with the back of his left hand. Those are the dried blood smears on his hands. Then he pulls out his handkerchief and holds it to his nose until he has staunched the flow. It wasn't a big hit, at first, only a light blow, with little blood flow. And that's it. That minor assault was the beginning of all this.'

I looked around. The police were following this closely. I could tell they all bought it. They, too, could see it happening the way I was describing it.

'He then crumples his handkerchief into a ball and stuffs it back into his trouser pocket, right where we found it. The other major facial injuries happened much later and certainly at a different place, almost certainly there at the chicken ranch.'

I continued with the autopsy. I could see that the mid-facial fractures and injuries were the crux of the assault. A complete understanding of what had happened could only be achieved by dissecting the face in layers, peeling aside skin and fat, then the layers of muscle, right down to bone. I wouldn't be able to stop there. I would then have to meticulously disarticulate and disassemble the fragmented delicate bones of the cheeks and the bony frame around the eyes. It would take hours or days to figure out the anatomical injuries that a few, furious seconds of violent kicking had inflicted. It would really add nothing to what I could already deduce.

But then I had a thought. I might be able to short-cut this process, after all.

'Pat, can you organise a CAT scan of the head and neck before we start?'

This was a bit innovative. CAT scans in autopsies are routine now in many centres, and with virtually all types of autopsy, but they weren't at all common back then in 2007.

I had to ask the radiologist on call, my friend John Goulden, to come in over the weekend to do this one and he agreed with his characteristic good grace. He was actually very interested in what there was to see.

'Pretty severe mid-facial trauma,' he explained, pointing at the display screen in the darkened CAT suite. Stinson's body lay sealed in a thick, leak-proof plastic body bag, entirely enclosed by the arch of the scanner. The machinery circled and thudded around the bag, shining the piercing rays that revealed the deeply hidden inner injuries. One advantage of doing CAT scans on the dead is that they don't have to be told not to move. I guess the radiation exposure becomes unimportant, too.

'There's posterior displacement of both maxillae and zygomatic arches. The brain is swollen with subarachnoid haemorrhages and there are petechial haemorrhages into the brain cortex,' John told me.

His description was dispassionate and technical as he looked at the dehumanised black-and-white X-ray images, but he and I could both see that this was medically horrific. These were massive, grotesque and non-survivable injuries.

John's assessment was spot on. I knew that, because I had seen the reality that was currently concealed by the bright-blue body bag lying on the scanner's inner table.

Pat and I wheeled the trolley back through the deserted hospital corridors and took the lonely lift just to the left of the main passage leading to the hospital cafeteria. Few people passing by on their way to their morning coffee and muffins know why there's a single lift in that particular place. There may be other reasons, for all I know, but I know for sure that it's the means by which the dead from anywhere in the hospital come down, lying horizontally on the gurney that takes them to their final port of departure.

Back in the mortuary, I continued to carry out my examination. The CAT scan was revealing, but there was more evidence to find. As I dissected the neck, I discovered his larynx was shattered. His Adam's apple (as the larynx, or voice box, is colloquially known) was split vertically down the middle, there was bleeding into and around it, and his hyoid bone was fractured. A hyoid bone fracture usually causes gasps of horror from doctors, as this is a classical sign of manual strangulation. I didn't think a manual strangulation was part of the assault. Given the way the other injuries were inflicted in that final, frenzied attack, it was clear to me that the killer had put his boot in and jumped on the victim's throat with all his weight in order to create this hellish constellation of injuries.

An assault on the face is usually a sign of pure, distilled anger. A concentration on the eyes is always from hatred and loathing. A crushing of the airway unequivocally signifies the intention to cause death. All these hateful elements were there.

'Look at this!' I exclaimed.

I had carefully snipped the bladder open, because I wanted to collect some urine to test for alcohol and drugs of abuse. Everyone crowded around and looked into the bladder.

There was the corrugated, pinkish lining of the bladder sac — and nothing else.

'Bugger all there,' said Pat. Everyone looked at me, puzzled.

'Exactly. Not a drop of urine at all. Not even a millilitre. So where is it?' I looked around at the watchful faces. Their expressions were still blank.

'I seem to remember that your body produces a millilitre

of urine a minute. And there is absolutely none in here. I don't think that's possible.'

I thought a moment.

'There are a couple of possibilities, I suppose. He could have emptied his bladder there by the gate just before being murdered. Or maybe he pissed his pants when they killed him. I would guess that would be more likely.'

Pat went and pulled the underwear and denims out of their bag and examined the crotch of both to see if they were sodden. He shook his head.

'Dry as a bone. Not even damp. Both of them. He hasn't pissed himself.'

'Surely it would be odd for the murderer or murderers to let him quietly piss there in front of them, and then go on afterward and beat him to death in a red rage? Usually murders are uncontrolled, violent, rapid things. Murderers don't tend to be so accommodating as that.'

I was thinking, and now that I had heard he was an active paedophile, other scenarios were starting to suggest themselves to me.

'There's another possibility, of course. Has he been held imprisoned somewhere else, maybe locked up for a few days? And given nothing to eat or drink so he's become dehydrated? He wouldn't have any urine then.'

The detectives listened politely but I could see they were pretty sceptical. Interesting theory, their expressions said, but there's no evidence. And, anyway, get real. This is Palmerston North. We provincials just aren't that sophisticated when we commit crimes.

Then I remembered his eyeball electrolytes. Both eyes showed he was in a normal state of hydration at the second he died. No dehydration there at all, and he even had plenty of glucose on board, so no starvation, either. Bugger. Drop that theory. I clammed up and thankfully no-one ever brought it up again. But I did check my memory about the rate of production of urine and what an empty bladder might mean. I called John Chrisp. John is a very well-informed urological surgeon. He would know the answer. His cell phone rang for some time before he answered. I put the problem to him.

'We always see the ureters spurting small amounts of urine into the bladder during operations, so yes, it's a continuous flow. Your one millilitre a minute seems about right. But I'll check and email you.'

'Thanks, John. That's really helpful.'

There was quite a bit of background noise. I thought I could hear glasses clinking. That seemed incongruous for this early on a Sunday morning so I wondered what he was doing.

'Sorry to disturb you,' I said. 'I hope you're having a peaceful Sunday at home?'

'Actually, no,' John laughed. 'I'm in Rome on holiday. We're just having a bottle of wine with dinner.'

Oops again. Cell-phone technology has shrunk the world.

* * *

It didn't take the police long to re-trace the last hours of Stinson's life. There had been a party at a house in Andrew Avenue in Palmerston North that Friday night. Stinson was there. He wasn't actually personally invited, but was there as the partner of his current paramour of the previous three months, who lived there, too. It's not clear whether she or any of the folk in the house were aware of Stinson's past. Probably not, I would guess. For in addition to the four pending charges for which he was on bail, he'd been convicted of indecent assault in 1967 as a 17-year-old and had five further convictions, all on girls under the age of 16, between 1974 and 1984. It's not the kind of background you look for in your perfect party guest — if you knew about it.

Sleeping in a room upstairs in Andrew Avenue was the ten-year-old daughter of a young mother who had been taken in and given sanctuary in the house, after herself suffering a dreadful sexual attack in Waikanae. During the party, the young mother went upstairs to check on her daughter, just as good mothers always do.

She came upon Stinson raping her daughter on his lap.

That something like this would happen was probably predictable when Stinson was released on bail. The ending, too, was now all but inevitable.

'It sounded like they were having a party and there were a few people around,' a neighbour said. 'Then all of a sudden I heard all this yelling and it sounded like a fight and this woman started screaming. I heard someone running and then I heard more people run out and jump into a couple of cars and drive off.' He didn't hear anyone return.

Police soon arrested Bruce Tamatea, 46, and Aubrey Harrison, 27, as well as the girl's young mother. The details were revealed in court and they pretty well matched the events as we had already deduced them from the scene and the autopsy. Stinson was bundled into a car and they drove into the night.

'I thought they were taking him for a ride to scare him. I don't think they could make up their minds where they wanted to go. By then I just wanted to go home and forget the whole thing.'

The young mother said she hit him at the house and again in the car. He sustained a lightly bloodied nose from those blows, which would explain the older dried blood on his hands and the handkerchief.

They pulled up outside the chicken ranch.

He was indeed permitted to piss at the gates of the ranch, so that explained the complete absence of urine that I had found. To kill in cold blood is hard. I think they watched him pissing and vulnerable and used the moment to steel themselves and whip themselves into a frenzy of outrage at what he had done.

'I was in a rage,' the young mother said. 'I kicked him in the face. I said: "You're a filthy piece of shit." He said: "I'm sorry. I'm sorry." He was crying and saying: "I'm sorry for what I did." It wasn't enough. I wanted more. I just froze and stood there. I just watched the whole thing. They hit him on the head with a hammer and they stomped on his head. They stood on his throat. They just kept doing that till he stopped breathing.'

Bruce Tamatea took sole responsibility and pleaded guilty, saying he carried out the execution alone.

'They shouldn't be here,' he said, indicating his two co-accused. 'I killed Glen Stinson. It was only supposed to be a bash. I had the hammer. I used the hammer. I went too far. I kicked him till his eyes popped out.'

Justice Forrest Miller sentenced the pair of men to life imprisonment for murder with a minimum ten-year non-parole period for Tamatea and 12 years for Harrison. The vulnerable young mother was given three years for manslaughter. Bruce Tamatea was denied parole for the third time in September 2019 but has retired from the notorious Black Power gang and is making determined progress towards a release in the not too distant future.

Glen Stinson was apparently a charming gentleman, who had been married three times and had three children. He had a talent for worming his way into the trust and confidence of the families of his victims. He met his eldest son, who is also a sex offender, for the first time when they were both in Manawatu Prison.

Whenever I think of this case, I can't help feeling our system is pretty hopeless at dealing with paedophiles. No-one knows the cause of paedophilia, but I believe it is now recognised as a psychiatric disorder. In the most affected — and often the most publicised — cases, the perpetrator's behaviour is down to urges that are simply irresistible. The consequences, of course, are awful. There is, as I understand it, no cure for the disorder, but it seems to me that dealing with it in the criminal justice system with prison sentences and then a release on parole is pretty stupid.

We really need a better system, although I can't say what this would look like. It's way beyond anything a simple, jobbing provincial pathologist could ever devise.

Glen Ronald Stinson. 27 July 2007. Requiescat in pace.

CHAPTER 9

Shotguns in the Manawatu

There are plenty of shotguns in the Manawatu. More than there are rifles, for sure.

The opening of the duck-shooting season early in May starts a noticeable buzz of activity. Early in May, the ducks come to town. They settle in the Hokowhitu Lagoon and on The Square, where they squabble over the bread brought down by toddlers and children. Feeding them isn't really encouraged — it's even frowned upon — but we all do it with our children.

The ducks also throng the river bank on the city side. My Labrador chases them and they paddle into the safety of midstream, but usually no further. They avoid the far bank, which is way too close for comfort to the waterways, lakes and dams beyond. The birds have noted the activity in those areas, people decking their mai mais with camouflage. They know exactly what it means. It means the shotguns are coming out soon.

As I walk the dog by the river each morning during the duck-shooting season, we hear the distant blasts of the guns rolling in from the countryside. She pricks up her ears and whines as she gazes across the river, her atavistic desires calling her towards the sounds of the shoot.

With so many shotguns around, it's not surprising that pathologists see quite a bit of their effect on the human body.

Many of the wounds inflicted by shotguns are, of course, suicides. The easiest site for suicide victims to target is their own heads, usually through the temple, often between the eyes, but sometimes through the mouth or beneath the chin. The gun is designed to kill at a range of 40 to 50 metres. Its point-blank destructive power is just incredible.

A storm of fire and hot gases blows from the end of the barrel when the trigger is pulled, burning, singeing and clubbing the hairs, crisping the skin and staining it with soot and smoke. There can be an obvious circular brand burned into the skin where the explosive gases have ballooned it up onto the hot metal of the barrel. But it's what comes next that really does the damage. A phalanx of metal pellets and the plastic cup that contains them comes out of the cartridge at 800 miles per hour, bursts through the bone and into the soft grey and white matter of the brain. The expansion of the hot gases in the closed compartment of the skull virtually atomises the head, blowing it to bits.

I personally find these patients the hardest and most devastating to face of all the many, varied causes of death we have. There's just something about an explosive decapitation that is profoundly unnerving. I just feel sick at the first sight of them. 'Move!' I have to say to myself. 'Do it! Help them! Their trials are past. Yours aren't so bad in comparison.'

As you can imagine, the pattern of injuries changes quite quickly as you get further away from the weapon. There's a 90 per cent death rate up close, but this falls to just a few per cent out at 50 metres. The distance of the killer and their gun from the victim is important in murder investigations to work out the final scene at the moment the trigger is pulled.

Distance was important in the first homicide I ever investigated in the Manawatu. It was early April 1988 and I felt very important as I went down to the mortuary clutching the police report and the coroner's authority to carry out the autopsy under my arm. Things had been a lot less formal than this in Africa. There in Rhodesia, I never saw a police officer in the mortuary. Instead, I did an autopsy, filed a report and never heard another word. I suppose we were so overwhelmed with the multitude of distressed, live patients and war casualties that the police and judges and lawyers took pity on us and just let us get on with things.

Now, as I look back, though, to that day in 1988, it was a pretty basic investigation for a homicide. There was no team of CIB detectives, no briefing about the scene and circumstances, and I don't recall any photographers. I think there was just Bruce Scott, the chief mortuary assistant, myself and our patient, Bruce Barclay, who was lying on a shining gurney in a spotless mortuary.

We always said you could eat your breakfast off a floor that Bruce Scott had cleaned.

The naked body lying in the mortuary was that of a muscular 30-year-old man in his prime, with a horrific, gaping hole in the left side of his neck.

'Christ!'

I couldn't help but recoil a bit. I had seen much, much worse in Africa, but somehow it was surprising here in this freezing room of death in the New Zealand autumn. Thank

God we live in a society where even the pathologists can still find a violent death a shocking exception rather than the rule.

Bruce Barclay was an unemployed welder from Takaro in Palmerston North. A lot of folk were unemployed in those days in the provinces in New Zealand. The whole place was a bit shabby. Britain had ditched us for Europe a decade before, and the effect of a host of bad economic policies had since come home to roost as well. Barclay was associated with the Mothers Motorcycle Club. It would be my guess that he had been out drinking with his mates that night, but I didn't measure his blood-alcohol level, which would certainly be routinely done these days. They had continued to drink in the club's pad hidden by a high, corrugated-iron fence out on the Napier Road. One of his mates had apparently produced a shotgun at midnight and Bruce, here, was the product of what followed.

His throat was a tragic hole from front to back under his left jaw. Everything was gone — skin, muscle, carotid arteries, jugular vein and so many important nerves that it is beyond my powers to name them all. They had all vanished in an explosion of lead and hot gases.

I was scared. I had better get this right. What will a New Zealand court want to know, anyway? I got to work. My first task was to discover at what range the shot had been fired.

There was no burning, no soot, and no powder around the wound. Not point-blank, then, I thought, and more than 30 centimetres. That's something, anyway.

'Look here,' I said to Bruce Scott. He looked at our patient's neck reluctantly. He was of an older generation of assistant.

We respected him not only for his fanatical diligence when it came to hygiene, but also for his Trojan work ethic. His philosophy was to just get on and do his own job well, not to get involved with someone else's problems.

'The skin is scalloped around the edges. It's not a perfect circle. That means the pellets were beginning to spread out. That's about a metre's range, you see? The further away, the greater the scalloping. This is just starting.'

Bruce nodded, more out of politeness than anything. He'd already worked for a number of pathologists and was no doubt used to our oddities. I could tell he wasn't terribly interested. He was receiving information that he clearly regarded as well above his pay grade.

I searched through the pulverised flesh, tugging the tissue with my forceps until a portion pulled away and allowed me to extract two separate bits of the wad, sodden and still reeking of explosive, from within the hole.

'I knew this would be in here! The wad follows the pellets for about one and a half metres and then falls to the ground at about two metres. The wad had to be somewhere in here. So the range is between one and one and a half metres.'

Barclay's mouth was filled with an unpleasant mess of masticated, battered fish, which added to the generally poor impression that his stained and carious teeth and his gums, swollen with gingivitis, made. I slit the back of the oesophagus open with my scissors down to the stomach. A bolus of fish was stuck halfway down his gullet.

'Caught there like a time capsule!' I said. 'One second he's swallowing his fish and then, Bang! He's dead and the fish is caught there forever, suspended in mid-passage. I guess it proves there wasn't a physical fight going on when he was shot. It's pretty difficult to eat, swallow and fight all at the same time.'

I can't remember much about the trial, though I was surprised that a not-guilty verdict was returned, very quickly, by the jury. The police called in to see me one morning shortly afterwards. Detective Constable White sat comfortably in my office and told me the events of that night.

'Barclay and his mates had been out on the piss since early evening and just before midnight they picked up fish and chips and went to a place on the Napier Road. There was an argument and his mate grabbed a shotgun and pointed it at Barclay. Apparently Barclay ignored him and carried on eating his fish. He mocked him, saying, "You'd never pull that trigger." That was the end of it. This was all witnessed by another of his friends, Angel Moondust.'

It was all pretty tawdry, really. A petty argument, too much drink, a gang culture and a shotgun is all it takes. A life is simply blasted out of existence. Pretty pathetic, but this is how a significant part of our society lives.

Professionally, I was pleased with my efforts. For once, all the pathology findings fitted the scene perfectly and the shotgun and shell had all read the books and behaved exactly as predicted.

Bruce Lindsay Barclay. 4 April 1988. Requiescat in pace.

* * *

I always enjoy the Waitangi Day holiday. It's placed in a good spot, a break to ease the passage out of the silly period of Christmas and New Year and not quite yet into the working year. In 2002, the holiday fell on a Wednesday, so the week was further divided into two sets of two short working days, which is even better than usual. We had settled down for a family day by the pool and I was just firing up the barbecue to start lunch when the police called.

I wasn't too worried. It was already late morning so nothing much could happen for the rest of the day. Famous last words.

'Gidday, Doc. We have a situation in Highbury.'

'Situation'. That was a new one to me. 'Suspicious scene', yes. 'Homicide', yes. But a 'situation'?

'There's a body at an address in Coventry Street. Male juvenile, probably shot and hidden in the yard. We need you to have a look and see what you think. And can you do the Life Extinct certificate while you're there?'

That was unusual, too. Today was proving a day of firsts. All the bureaucratic work like Life Extinct papers was usually done before I arrived. Dr Jack Drummond, the police surgeon, rarely missed a significant event such as a shooting and he always smoothed away all this preliminary paperwork.

'Of course I can. But why hasn't the police doctor on call been?'

'That's because of the situation here. We've closed off the area because this is gang-related. The Mongrel Mob and Black Power are facing each other off. We've got armed police keeping them apart but it's pretty tense over there.'

So that was it, then. Gang warfare. A 'situation' indeed. Should be a doddle. Or maybe not.

I resigned myself to a day back in the harness and loaded up my car. I was driving a 17-year-old Daihatsu Charade at the time, which my children called Pinocchio, and quite frankly it was stuffed. There were blotches of rust peeking through the wings and the bonnet was a faded pink, contrasting oddly with the otherwise red car, the result of years of throwing buckets of boiling water over it in the depths of icy winter mornings. Pinocchio just would not fire up without that starting bucket. Elayne had discovered the technique. I was sceptical at first, but, God only knows how or why, it always worked.

Pinocchio and I crossed town and rolled up Coventry Street.

In front of me, about halfway down and blocking the entire road, were the red and black backs of dozens of patched members of Black Power. Their body language oozed aggression. The atmosphere was like a fuse: one spark and it would explode.

I was pulling over and stopping just behind them and wondering whether I might have made a terrible mistake. There wasn't a police car in sight. Angry warrior faces were turning towards me, registering disbelief at my car. I wondered whether I shouldn't just slap Pinocchio in reverse and high-tail it home. But it was too late for that.

I climbed out, pulling my bag behind me. A host of faces were glaring at me and they weren't friendly, I can tell you. Three gang members walked stiffly up to me, like dogs with their hackles raised.

'What do you want?' This wasn't a friendly inquiry, either.

'I'm the pathologist. A doctor. I've been called to see someone who has been killed.'

I felt nervous as a kitten. This was no place for a skinny white boy like me to be, for sure.

'Ah, a doctor.' He nodded his understanding, but his expression didn't soften. 'Come through. It's the doctor!' he called out to the watching men. He made a gesture waving the cordon open. 'Come through,' he repeated. The hostility was still there, but it had swung like a torch beam back towards some target to their front. Ludicrously, it occurred to me that I had forgotten to lock my car. Should I go back and do it now? The gang might take offence and God knows they were offensive enough already. So I left it.

Through the cordon I went. I couldn't believe my eyes.

There was a small group of two or three armed police in front of the milling horde. I had never seen nor had I ever expected to see police dressed like this in New Zealand. It was as though I had stumbled into a Darth Vader party: black ballistic vests, sinisterly shaped Kevlar helmets, communication mouthpieces and audio connections, and professionally cradled Bushmaster carbines. All in black. The blackest possible black.

'In Palmerston North?' I marvelled. 'Really?'

Somewhere out there beyond the Black Power horizon seethed the Mongrel Mob, transmitting back hatred and warning. You could almost feel it. The tiny Armed Offenders Squad seemed little enough to hold the line of civilisation and order.

'Thanks for coming, Doc. Sorry to get you out on a holiday.'

The conventionally dressed CIB detective clearly hadn't been invited to the Darth Vader party. His voice was relaxed and conversational. It was a weird contrast to the emotional thunderstorm crackling in the Highbury sky that day. He briefed me at the roadside before leading me towards number

26, the angry ranks of Black Power looking on. As we walked, we were joined by one or two other police officers.

'A gunshot was reported to us earlier this morning. We sent out a patrol but found nothing. That shot must have been it, about 0200 this morning. Nothing much goes on around here come early morning but he was spotted at 11.15 by a David Dawson across there at number 35. The body is hidden in the yard under a bush, as you'll see.'

'Hidden? You mean someone put him there?'

'Doesn't look like it. More like he went there himself. You'll see what I mean.'

'What's the gang connection? Why are they so rarked up?'

The detective shrugged. 'We reckon this is Wallace Whatuira. Only 16 years of age. He's a Black Power prospect and his uncle is John Whatuira, head of the local Black Power. This area also has quite a few known Mongrel Mob addresses nearby. I guess he was just in the wrong place at the wrong time.'

'And met the wrong people,' I added. 'Let's go and have a look at young Wallace.'

It was sad. There was a simple, suburban bungalow and a yard with not much of a garden scratched out, a few scraggly bushes here and there. Pretty typical for this street. Crouched by the side of the fence, partly hidden by a bush, was a body, still upright, his head leaning forward on his left wrist as though he were asleep. A small knapsack lay beside him. I knelt before him and examined him.

'Shotgun,' I said to the detectives. They already knew. It was obvious. There was a spread of pellets across his entire front chest and down as far as his waist. His right arm was also hit. Bloodstaining was clear on his clothes, but it was light.

'I agree with you,' I said. 'He's hidden himself away and quietly died as he crouched here. It doesn't look as though it was quick, but I suppose the perpetrator was still out there so he had to lie doggo and couldn't get to help.'

The detective nodded. 'When will you do the post-mortem? We've still got a bit to do here. And then there's that lot. God knows when they'll settle down.' He gestured towards the battle lines. 'Reinforcements are coming in from around the district, but we're a bit stretched at the moment.'

'Tomorrow morning at 9 a.m., okay?'

'We'll be there.'

The solid phalanx of gang members shuffled apart to let me through. They seemed less threatening to me now, different somehow. I thought I heard a few respectful murmurs, too, as I slowly edged through them. More likely I was so inconsequential that they didn't really even see me.

Pinocchio was waiting close by, quite untouched. Of course he was. I would wager he was the most secure car anywhere in Palmerston North that day.

* * *

Wallace Whatuira was hit 245 separate times by shotgun pellets. That is the number of separate entry holes that I counted. They were arranged in a scattered pattern across his chest and abdominal wall as well as over his right arm. The average density over his trunk was one pellet per five square centimetres, which is roughly the size of a postage stamp. There was a pellet for every 15 square centimetres on his right arm, which is roughly the size of a matchbox. That's an awful lot of lead coming in. The density made it clear that he was hit full-on by the shot, which indicated that it was deliberate. This was no accidental blow winging an innocent bystander.

'What do you reckon about the range, Doc?' The CIB detectives were predictable. The same old questions. They knew the answers just as well as I did, the same old answers.

'Here' — I pointed to Wallace's body — 'there is no cavitating injury or burn marks, no mark of the wad hitting him, so this is distant. How distant? Well, I use Bernard Knight's formula, which is pretty good for a conventional, unchoked, unmodified shotgun.' Without meaning to, I was using the words that I would use on my day in court, when I faced the lawyers' probing questions. The formula in question was devised by the legendary Welsh professor of forensic pathology, Sir Bernard Knight. The detectives were familiar with it, and some of them probably knew it well enough to know that according to it, one-third of the spread of the pellets in centimetres equals the range of fire in metres.

I picked up a tape measure and extended it across Wallace's body, over the hundreds of blood-blebbed puncture wounds. I measured from the top of the chest to the bottom of the lower abdomen, and then from the left side of the chest to the border of the right arm.

'Hold the arm out a little from the body. As if he was standing upright and carrying his knapsack by his side. I'm trying to get the most natural position his arm would have been in. I mean, he clearly wasn't squashed up like this on a gurney out there on Coventry Street or wherever it was, was he?'

With his arm away from his side, it was clear the pellets had spread a similar distance in all directions. I measured the area hit at 47 by 43 centimetres.

'I make that 14 to 15 metres' firing range. So he wasn't that close.'

Close or not, what had the pellets done to Wallace's insides?

The shotgun is a lethal weapon, make no mistake. That's why it was used by the Americans as their weapon of choice in trench warfare in 1918. And that's why, that same year, the Kaiser felt he had to declare it an inhumane weapon and therefore forbidden by the 1907 Hague Convention. Not that this declaration made a jot of difference: the Yanks just carried on using it, anyway.

Both Wallace's lungs were punctured. The right lung had collapsed and was surrounded by one and a half litres of blood pushing the heart way over into the left chest cavity. A pellet had punctured the pericardial sac around the heart, and there were six pellets embedded in the surface of the heart itself. One had even penetrated to damage the valves deep within.

As if these fatal injuries were not enough, there were perforations to each and every part of his bowel, all survivable singly, but in aggregate, they were horrific. The liver was punctured 18 times and there was even more free blood lying within the abdomen. That made at least a third of his blood volume leaking from a hundred different puncture sites and sloshing uselessly within body cavities. With his lung capacity halved and his heart battered by a storm of pellets, it was surprising he'd managed to run as far and hide as he did.

The full story of Wallace's last night did come out in time.

That Tuesday night, he and four Black Power mates had decided to take a shortcut down Cowley Place to a mate's house in Botanical Road. They knew that Cowley Place harboured a Mongrel Mob hangout, but they went anyway. It was a fatal decision. A member of the Mob spotted them as they passed by. A chase began.

'It's the mutts! Move it!' Wallace and his friends began running.

They weren't fast enough.

One of the Black Power gang who was ambushed on that street with Wallace told what happened next. He knew the names of their pursuers. One was his uncle, Leon Hakaraia. He also recognised Andrew Popo and John Waara, amongst others.

'As the mutts were approaching us, they were saying: "C'mon, niggers" and barking. Leon ran up to John and Andrew and in between them ... As he did this, he jumped in the air and fired from chest height ... His scarf fell down off of his face. He fired one shot. I didn't recognise the firearm but saw the sparks as it was fired. I didn't see him carrying anything until he arrived at this point.'

That flash and the bang was the first indication of what they were facing. It was serious before. Now it was lethal. They ran for their lives. Two of them ran up a long drive and hid in the back seat of a car, covering themselves up with a blow-up toy castle that was lying there.

'We were freaked out. I thought they might come after us, after me.'

Despite his terrible injuries, Wallace managed to race clear, making 200 metres before hunkering down behind his bush in Coventry Street.

The witness's recall was so precise, and it tied up so neatly with what I had found, that I imagined the court case would be straightforward. With such damning eyewitness evidence, the defendants might plead guilty. I might not even be called.

A depositions hearing was arranged over a couple of days so that the evidence could be examined to establish whether the three Mongrel Mob members had a case to answer. All three had already been locked up for the past four months in Manawatu Prison, waiting for this day in court. It was all on. The ducks were all in a row.

But there was a surprise in store for us all when the 16-year-old witness was called.

'The details are all wrong,' he said, when asked to comment on the signed statement he had given to the police.

'Which part of it is wrong?' Mathew Downs, who was the Crown prosecutor, asked patiently.

'All of it.'

'Have you forgotten who was there? Who fired the gun?'

'Yes. We were all drunk.'

That was that. It lasted only an hour.

Leon Tuirirangi Hakaraia walked free. He had beaten a murder rap against all expectation.

The witness's mother put it well, when she was asked why her son had 'forgotten' what had happened that night.

'He must have got scared … I'm not angry. I'm just glad it's over. When I see him again, I'll give him a big hug. I hope he stays away from gangs, now.'

We could, alas, deliver no justice for Wallace, no matter how strong the evidence. 'The investigation is not so much unsolved as unresolved,' was how Detective Inspector Doug Brew put it.

Leon Hakaraia remained a member of the Mob, serving the odd jail sentence here and there. Some years later,

Andrew Popo was sentenced to eight years and nine months for running down and killing Sergeant Derek Wootton as he laid road spikes to stop the car in which Popo was racing away from the police. John Waara was locked up in solitary confinement in Manawatu Prison, where one night he was stabbed in both eyes with a fork. Both were horrifically gouged and damaged. No-one knows who or how: it's a mystery how anyone got at him in his secure cell. Waara didn't lay a complaint and absolutely refused to co-operate with the police. 'An eye for an eye, a tooth for a tooth, a life for a life', as the saying goes. It was widely believed that this was a revenge attack for Wallace. From this perspective, John Waara was fortunate not to lose his life.

Wallace Stanley Whatuira. 6 February 2002.
Requiescat in pace.

* * *

Some murders capture the public imagination and are endlessly analysed and luridly pulled apart in *The Herald*, in *The Dominion*, in *North & South* and at every media stop in between. We in the Manawatu have had perhaps more than our fair share of local examples. The murder in Palmerston North of Christine and Amber Lundy in 2001 was one of these. The killing of Scott Guy near Feilding was another. The murder itself was brutal enough to get people talking. But it was the trial and its outcome that ensured this crime would be speculated upon for years to come. I still get asked about this one more than any other. I will say at the outset that none of the pathologists in Palmerston North, including me, was involved in the investigation. I never saw the scene. I never examined Guy's body or saw any photographs, and I was never formally consulted on evidence. So, disappointingly, I can't reveal any secret background fact that isn't already publicly known. Justice has been done to the investigation in other books, particularly Mike White's *Who Killed Scott Guy?: The case that gripped a nation*, and this is not the place for the whole, long and complicated story.

The double gate to Scott Guy's property on Aorangi Road wasn't normally closed. But when Guy reached it early one Thursday morning in July 2010, he found it shut. He got out of his ute to open it and was gunned down as he did so. Guy, the victim, was young, blond and strikingly good-looking. The man who was soon charged with his murder was his dark and muscular brother-in-law, Ewen Macdonald. Their wives, Scott's sister Anna Guy (who was married to Ewen) and Scott's wife Kylee, were both beautiful women and together the four made an eye-catching, handsome pair of couples. But at the trial, sagas of jealousy between the brothers-in-law emerged, involving all sorts of nastiness — foul, anonymous letters; secret midnight 'missions' to do graffiti, commit arson and vandalism; deer poaching; the senseless slaughter of farm animals and (as if the taking of a young man's life wasn't enough) the slaughter of a litter of chocolate Labrador puppies. For most of the general public, the last atrocity was the clincher.

The trial of Ewen Macdonald had all the elements, and the high calibre of the counsel involved ensured it was pure theatre. Ben Vanderkolk led the prosecution and the charismatic Greg King the defence. The public loved it. Every day, there was frantic competition to grab a seat in the overflowing public gallery, and those who couldn't be at court followed the trial avidly in the media. Elayne and I were no exceptions.

Macdonald was eventually acquitted, largely because the Crown hung its case on a set of footprints found at the scene. They were made by dive boots, and the particular pair that the Crown insisted made them were way too small to fit Macdonald's feet. The gun was never found, although a shotgun was definitely used. Everyone in the Manawatu has a theory or a perspective on the crime. Mine is from a pathologist's perspective. From the first, I took a professional interest in the fatal injuries and what they might mean.

I watched Ben Vanderkolk presenting the Crown case on the TV One news and read about it in more detail in *The Dominion*. We heard that two shots were fired at Scott Guy. One was violently destructive into the right and centre of his neck. The other peppered his left hand, arm, the side of his face and sent pellets up through his cheekbones and eye sockets, into his brain.

'I wonder what the range they have decided on is,' I said to Elayne. 'That's important. They surely must have worked that out very carefully.'

As if on cue, the court reporter covering the day's evidence then told us.

'The Crown produced this shotgun, which they say could have been used in the murder — the blast fired from three or four metres away.'

The weapon shown was a two-shot 'under and over' Lanber shotgun, a popular duck-shooting tool. I could guess from this, and from the many subsequent written descriptions, what I would expect to see in a post-mortem on

Scott's body. Knowing the range, it would be a simple matter of applying the reverse of Sir Bernard Knight's formula, so that a range of three to four metres would produce a spread of pellets of nine to 12 centimetres. So I would expect to see pellet wounds scattered over that area on the left side of his face and his left arm and hand from that second shot. There would be no central hole and no wad or wad marks from this hit. That's straightforward.

So much for the scattered second set of injuries. What did the wound from the supposed first shot look like?

It was Scott Guy's neighbour, truck driver David Berry, who found Scott's body early that morning. 'There was a bit of blood around the shoulder and at the back,' Berry told the court. He saw a gaping wound in Guy's neck that a pathologist later measured at 13 centimetres across. Berry was sure that Guy's throat had been cut. According to the TV One news, 'not even the police knew that Scott Guy had been shot until they found the shotgun cartridge wadding in his neck'. That's what the reporter said. I was immediately sceptical of that claim, as the CIB hardly came down in the last shower. The police must have known long before the post-mortem that Scott had been killed by a shotgun, from the spread of pellets across his face and arm.

The interesting and critical fact to me is that the wadding was found buried in his neck wound. It was, of course, not an actual felt wad, as was used in old-fashioned shotgun cartridges to separate the pellets from the explosive charge, but a plastic shot cup or piston. It was this large plastic cup that was embedded in Scott's neck.

'The older wadding typically stops following the pellets at about a metre and a half away,' I explained to Elayne, who was pretending to listen to me while getting our tea ready. 'And then it drops to the ground at around two metres.'

The modern plastic cup behaves much like the old wad. It has side flaps that open out like the petals of a flower after discharge. The air-brake effect sees it decelerate and part company with the cloud of pellets it once contained at about a metre from the muzzle of the gun. Left to its own devices, the cup may still continue alone on its pathway for up to 30 metres. But it loses energy rapidly enough that it is unlikely to follow the pellets into a wound beyond about two metres' range. This means, in principle, that the shot to Scott Guy's throat must have been from up close, as the wad had followed the mass of pellets in and was still deeply embedded in the wound. The range was probably little more than a metre to a metre and a half away, at the most. We know it was no closer, as the pathologist didn't find any trace of the powder tattoo or muzzle burn that will accompany a wound inflicted at very close range.

So, for me, there were two different injury patterns, and the range of each shot has to be considered separately from the other. The wound to the left side of the face and arm seems to have been fired from between three and four metres' range. The neck shot was fired from a little less than half that distance.

According to the Crown, Guy 'was killed by a shotgun blast to his throat followed by a second shot to his face, hands and arms', as Ben Vanderkolk quietly but authoritatively stated in court. According to his theory of the case, the first shot was to the neck and the second was fired as Scott fell backwards, which is why it was less accurate and more spread out. The Crown also said that the killer then walked up to his body to make certain he was dead, judging from footprint evidence.

This was all theoretically possible. Scott's neck injuries were either instantly fatal or, at the very least, totally incapacitating. I doubt Scott could have staggered further backwards on his own feet to account for the difference in distance, and neither the Crown nor defence ever suggested that he might have. The Crown accounts for the range discrepancy between the two shots by postulating that he fell stiffly backwards. He was 1.7 metres tall. If the first shot was from 1.5 metres away, then the second shot fired at him as he fell would add another 1.5 metres. That would give a range of three metres from the shotgun muzzle. It fits with the general perception of how gunshots work. We've all seen it so often in Hollywood movies: blast the bad guy with your pump-action shotgun and you will hurl him backwards through a glass window a couple of feet away.

But like most forensic pathologists, I absolutely do not buy it. If a shot had the power to knock over a victim, then the physics say the gun would have to knock the shooter backwards, too. In fact, there are thousands of real-life films and modern recordings of people and game being shot with all manner of weapons, and in every case, the victims crumple quietly to the ground where they stand. I can tell you that the experimental firing of high-velocity military rounds from close up at volunteers wearing ceramic body armour creates no backward movement at all, even when they balance on one foot. That violent blast backwards just never happens: it's a myth. But courts and juries and the public are quite unimpressed by these facts. They prefer to believe what they have seen with their own eyes in the movies.

Shotguns in the Manawatu

I wonder whether the shots that killed Scott Guy could have been fired the other way around. I can imagine a plausible sequence in which the murder might have unfolded that differs from the Crown theory.

First, this was definitely a coldly planned ambush. It wasn't, as the defence suggested, the act of a burglar who had been surprised by Guy's sudden arrival and who fired in a panic. To start with, most burglars don't carry weapons at all, let alone unwieldy weapons like loaded shotguns. Why would a burglar have chosen to come sneaking around at an hour when most farmers are already up and about? Why would a burglar close the gate? Why would he wait 20 seconds or more for Scott to open both gates before firing in his 'blind panic'? And why would he fire two shots in sequence rather than both barrels at once, or bolt after firing one barrel only? It makes no sense.

I think the murderer deliberately closed the gate and waited. Scott drove up in his ute and stopped, puzzled. After a moment, he must have shrugged and climbed out, leaving the lights of the vehicle on and the engine running. He opened the right-hand gate first, as it was closest to the driver's side. He then opened the left-hand gate. It had sagged a bit, so it stuck. He had to lift it up over the hump and push it open. Then he started back around his vehicle to the driver's side.

The killer was waiting in the darkness out of the beam of the headlights, just to the side of the right-hand gate post.

Scott then saw or heard something that really alarmed him. He might have suddenly had a premonition, or he might have put two and two together. He might actually have seen his killer pointing the gun at him, from three metres' range. We'll never know which it was. Either way, he reacted by ducking away to his right and throwing up his left arm in an instinctive, protective gesture. The killer fired his first shot. A number of pellets missed and, together with the plastic shot cup, they flew into the dark beyond the passenger's side of the idling ute. The stray pellets were later found by forensic firearms expert Mike Walsh embedded in the fence and a tree, while the shot cup lay some metres away in the grass beside the fence.

Not all of the pellets missed. Those that struck home were scattered across Guy's left arm, hand and face. Pellets penetrated his skull through his eye sockets and entered his brain. If Scott was ducking away, the path of the pellets would be upwards through his face. That is what they were found to be, and this is why the Crown suggested he was falling when struck by this shot.

That first shot was enough to drop Scott to the ground. But the killer, who was intent on murder, needed to be sure he was dead. He walked up close to Guy and delivered the 'coup de grâce' — the mercy shot, as it is called when a hunter dispatches a wounded animal. That's why his footprints were found right beside the body. The muzzle of the gun would be a metre to a metre and a half from Guy's neck as he stood over him. At that range, the shot would rip the throat open just like a savage knife slash and leave the shot cup deep in the tissues of the neck. That's exactly how the wound looked to David Berry, and that's exactly where the pathologist found the wad.

I would also expect to see 'scalloping' of the wound edges if the shot was fired at a metre-and-a-half range. I've never seen this confirmed.

What difference does it make if the shots were fired in the reverse order, you might ask? I would answer that it makes all the difference in the world. It's the sequence you would expect in an execution-style killing, and speaks very much to the murderer's intent.

Only the murderer knows what really happened that morning. The killing range and pattern of spread can only ever be estimated by real-life test-firing with the actual gun, using the same degree of choke and the same ammunition. The gun used in Scott's murder has never been found. It may have been a short- or a long-barrelled shotgun with full or half choke and all would result in quite a different pattern of spread and a different story.

In the end, my theory is just more speculation based on second-hand reports. It doesn't extend as far as suggesting who the actual murderer was. Ewen Macdonald served a little over five years in prison for the vicious acts of vandalism and arson he committed against Scott Guy's property and farm animals, but was acquitted of Guy's murder. He is divorced from Anna but has since remarried and lives in Christchurch. No-one has ever been brought to justice for Scott's murder.

Scott Guy. 8 July 2010. Requiescat in pace.

CHAPTER 10

Unfortunate Deaths

'Good morning, Paddy. What have you got for me today?'

'Motorcycle accident,' my mortuary assistant replied, and then paused, as if striking exactly the right, offhand note. 'With decapitation. Clean as anything you ever saw.'

'That's unusual,' I replied. 'We don't see that every day. He must have been doing a hell of a speed.'

'Aye, it came off just like a guillotine,' Paddy agreed, with gloomy relish. 'He went through a deer fence. One of the strands just took his head off. I've got him out on the table here for you.'

I went over and looked. There on a gurney lay the body of a young man, tattooed all over with intricate and coloured designs. There wasn't much undecorated skin left. Both arms and forearms were misshapen, broken, shattered and emulsified. The tattooed skin was all that was keeping those bags of pulp and blood and fragmented bone together. The legs were much the same.

So far, much like any other motorcycle accident.

But sticking oddly from the pulpy trunk was the bony column of the neck. It stood up proudly from the trunk like a tower constructed of the bones of the cervical vertebrae. They were all stripped clean of tissue and were gleaming with an ivory hue. There was no head attached.

The head lay beside the body on the gurney where Paddy had placed it. It was dark, acne-scarred and heavily tattooed to match the body. The facial tattoos, too, were of intricate and interesting designs that spoke of many hours' suffering. The only part that jarred was a social message on the forehead: 'FUCK THE POLICE' it said.

'I'm guessing he'd have a pretty uncomfortable time if he fell into the hands of the police,' I murmured quietly to myself.

Compared with the body, the head was relatively intact. A small, superficial split on the lower lip was all there was to see, despite the abrupt way in which it had parted company with the neck. As I set it down, my examination complete, the phone rang.

Paddy answered. 'Yes,' he said. 'Yes!' again, but louder.

I looked at him questioningly.

'The police are here to see you, Doctor,' he announced formally, almost as if he were some sort of butler.

'What do they want?'

The mortuary doorbell rang loudly to announce that someone had opened the door. We had put this in after a member of the public looking for the Audiology Department had wandered in during an autopsy. It must have seemed a scene from Hell. God only knows what lasting psychological effect this had left on him. I just hoped he was okay. Thank God the press didn't get to hear of it.

The Quick and the Dead

This time, it was two uniformed constables.

'Good morning,' I said. 'So what brings Her Majesty's constabulary into our humble mortuary?'

'We've come to tell you what happened with this bloke,' one said, smiling wickedly as he gestured at the body on the table.

'Well, what happened?'

'It's pretty odd, I can tell you.' He nodded at his companion. 'Tell the doctor what happened.'

'Well, we were on patrol up State Highway 1 when we saw the skid marks on the road from the motorcycle. We followed them for about 250 metres, so we reckon he was probably doing something like one-fifty kilometres per hour. Maybe even more. We found the bike in the ditch, but no sign of the rider. We searched up and down the road, in the ditch and the paddock next door. Nothing to find. We thought he might have been picked up by a passing car and taken to hospital. Or maybe he'd been uninjured and wandered off to look for help under his own steam. It took a while to find him on the far side of the road. He was ahead of the bike. That's why we missed him, at first. We only spotted him because I saw the deer fence up ahead looked buggered and I went to have a look. The body was on the other side of the road next to the fence hidden in the long grass. But the head had come off. That was a bit of a bugger, but eventually we found it on the other side of the fence in the paddock. About a kilometre back down State Highway 1, there was a house standing by itself. No neighbours anywhere. We decided to go back and ask if they'd heard or seen anything. A couple of hundred metres back along the road, I spotted something white lying partly hidden by grass at the side of the road. We pulled over to have a dekko. It was a dog, a white and black blotched dog, some sort of half-breed mutt. Bit of sheepdog, I reckon, and a lot of mongrel. About medium size, maybe 20 kilos or so. But it was dead. Head twisted. Neck at a funny angle, fresh blood running from the nose. It was still floppy. No stiffening. Freshly dead, then, I reckon.'

'You think he might have hit the dog and come off?'

'Yep, I reckon. Wouldn't take much to do it at that speed. So I pick the dog up by its tail and we go up to the house. It's pretty run-down, even by country standards. Paintwork gone, spouting hanging loose, cladding pretty well shot. A window boarded up. In the yard there's a pen with a pig scratching its arse on a post. I knock. We hear someone inside, but it still takes a couple of minutes. The door opens a crack and there's this rat-faced bloke, mouthful of crooked teeth, stinking of tobacco and piss. "What do youse want?" he says. So I hold up the dog in front of me by the tail. Blood's dripping from its nose onto the front step. Not that you'd notice any difference, because the whole place was crappy anyway. Never been cleaned in years, I'd say. "This your dog?" I ask him. He looks at us suspiciously. "So what if it is?" So I tell him the dog may have caused a fatal accident. Does he know anything about it? Then, get this, Doc. He opens the door, steps out, grabs the dog by its tail, turns, swings it a few times and hurls it over the fence into the bush next door. He then turns his back on us, goes inside and slams the door. Didn't say a bloody word at all. Yep. That was about it.'

'That's all?' I was fascinated. 'What'd you do?'

'We didn't think we'd get anything useful out of him. So we left.'

It seemed unbelievable.

'Is he going to be charged or anything?'

'What for? No proof, really, so what would we charge him with? We don't even know for sure whose dog it was. So it's just an accident, really.'

'Have you told Graham Hubbard?'

Graham was the coroner for the Manawatu district.

'Yep, we told him yesterday. He just smiled and said: "What an extraordinary reaction!"'

Later, as I completed the autopsy, I heard Paddy singing as he stroked his mop across the floor, sluicing bloodied water towards the drain.

'Go on Blue you good dog you
'Go on Blue you good dog you
'Blue laid down and died like a man
'Blue laid down and died like a man
'Now he's treein' possums in the promised land.'

'What's that?' I asked.

'What's what?'

'The song you're humming.'

'Oh, that. It's called "Old Dog Blue". By a guy called Jim Jackson.'

* * *

I first came across high-speed death in Africa, as the consequence of the crash of a jet. They're not a common sight for any pathologists to come across professionally, and you couldn't with any precision say that I or any other doctor really saw this one, either. The civil war in what would become the new state of Zimbabwe was at its height in 1979. A Canberra bomber was hit by a surface-

Unfortunate Deaths

to-air missile and was seen to fly off towards the sparsely populated hinterland of Mozambique with one wing hanging low like an injured bird. Somewhere out there, it flew uncontrolled and at high speed into the ground with a load of alpha bombs on board. This was a nasty piece of ordnance, a metal sphere designed to strike the ground, bounce and burst at a height of about six metres, spraying fragments and ball bearings over the immediate vicinity, rather like an outsized grenade. The Canberra was carrying several of them, and needless to say, the explosion when it hit the ground was immense.

A rescue team went in, but came back empty-handed.

'We reached the site,' they told us. 'There was fuck-all left. Absolutely no bloody trace of any bodies.' All they found was a smoking hole and part of an engine. I thought that was completely predictable.

My commanding officer, Bryan Knight, was enraged at this. He had shared a mess with the missing pilot.

'Chopper me in there!' he ordered the base commander. 'I'll find you a body! The families need something, anything — even just a finger to bury to know it is over! I will find them. Just let me go.'

It wasn't really rational and it was never going to happen. It was just too dangerous. The two crew, Kevin Peinke and JJ Strydom, were doubtless scattered across the bushveld and would never come home.

This episode was long out of my mind in late October 1989 when I got a call from the Air Force base at Ohakea, just south-west of Bulls.

'Gidday. Len Bagnell here.' Len was one of the RNZAF doctors at Ohakea Base Hospital. 'We've had an accident out here. Two Skyhawks have collided over the runway and one has gone in just beyond the 27 Runway threshold.'

'No!' I was stunned. 'Did the pilots manage to get out?'

'One managed to land okay but the plane's badly damaged. The second went in and exploded on impact.'

'Very sorry to hear that. I'm guessing the pilot didn't have time to eject?'

Why else would they phone us?

'It's a really long shot. We can't find a body. The eyewitnesses say the collision was forceful and the pilot may not have been conscious. Or he may even have been dead already. The altitude of the aircraft and the length of time she kept flying should have been enough for the pilot to eject. No-one saw that happen, but who knows? We can't find any trace of the body. Can you come and help us?'

'Of course,' I said. We would do whatever we could.

My assistant James and I raced out to Ohakea in my Daihatsu Charade. The gate guard was expecting us and the boom was smartly raised as we drove through. I parked Pinocchio outside the hospital and we met Len and a colleague. The facts were given to us briefly.

'They were a four-man formation from the Kiwi Red aerobatic team. They were tasked to practise aerobatics as they're due to perform at the Nissan Mobil 500 Race in December and for the opening of the Commonwealth Games next January. The two were peeling off for a "roll-under break" to land and it seems that Red 4 — that's NZ 6210 — didn't quite complete his roll and was hit by NZ 6211. The second Skyhawk managed to land but Red 4 plunged into the ground and exploded. That's about all we know, at this stage.'

Unfortunate Deaths

I later learned that this manoeuvre involved each of the aircraft in sequence, starting with the leader, rolling and turning beneath but in front of the following team members. At those speeds the tolerances were fine. The Australian Air Force would only do this display by reversing the order so the last aircraft led the way, each turning below and behind the flight path. Not so dramatic perhaps, but surely safer than turning in front of oncoming traffic.

We climbed into a vehicle and were driven through the base and out to where a cluster of vehicles was parked around the end of the runway. We joined a group of men who were standing, staring at the ground. Wreckage lay all about. A yellow-and-red chequered warning flag fluttered from a flagpole driven into the ground close by.

There was a large crater, maybe four feet deep. It lay centred on a two-strainer fence separating the aerodrome from a farm paddock. Twenty metres along, there was a gate leading into the field. The newly disturbed soil in the crater was loose and the adjacent grass was charred. There was only a light scatter of aluminium confetti within to show that an aircraft had dug this crater. Amongst the surrounding debris, I saw a distorted piece of sheeting bearing the blue roundel with its central red kiwi, a poignant symbol of our loss.

'There's not much to see in here,' an Air Force officer said. 'We think there may be some remains but we're not sure. Poor Crater.'

I glanced down into the crater, puzzled. It was much like any other hole in the ground, so far as I could tell.

'How do you mean? What's wrong with it?'

The officer looked at me and James. It was his turn to be puzzled.

'Flying Officer Graham Carter,' he said. 'His nickname was Crater.'

Despite the dreadful circumstances, I had to smile. It was nominative determinism at its best. How did they know?

I looked beyond the impact site. The engine had been flung away and lay alone further along the fence. A jagged, twisted wing with its aileron had been ripped off the fuselage and stood upright, its wingtip driven into the earth, some distance further still.

Everything spoke of a massive explosion.

We sifted through the crater and its surrounds. It took us a long while. Nothing I looked at resembled even the smallest fragment of tissue that would herald the end of our desperate search for Graham.

Then a policeman called to us.

'Can you come and have a look over here, Doctor? We may have found something.'

We made our way through the gate and into the farm paddock. There, a full 60 metres from the impact site, was a fragment of tissue. I picked it up gently and turned it over. James and I studied it carefully.

'It's partly burnt tissue isn't it?' I asked.

'Definitely.' James nodded. 'But it's not necessarily human, of course.'

'More over here, Doctor!' The policeman and an airman had moved on a further seven metres, even further from the impact point.

This find set any doubts to rest, for here was a right ear. And further on there was a portion of skull, too.

I felt sadness welling up as we reported that Flying Officer Graham 'Crater' Carter had been found. Of course, they knew all along he must be dead, but given the slightest chance, hope will linger even when it is quite irrational. It's a sadness that I often feel in the presence of the dead, particularly when the person is young and vibrant and has been killed so unexpectedly.

James arranged for a team to spread out and cover every inch of the field. It was a more complex task than simply collecting parts and putting them all in a pile in a body bag. The exact position of each part has to be meticulously documented. Then, later, we would examine each part individually to decide what it was. The usual system in aircraft accidents was to lay out lines in a numbered grid pattern to map the entire fall-out area, but that wasn't necessary in this instance. We used the paddock fence posts which were uniformly spaced seven metres apart as our reference line. The posts were numbered 1 to 35. The impact site was right on post 4. As each body part was found, its distance in relation to the nearest post and at right angles from the fenceline was measured and the body part was bagged with a number for that location.

Eighteen separate bags were collected and James painstakingly worked through each one identifying the tissue fragments, checking for disease and mapping their distribution. It took two days, a long and heart-rending task, but we were determined to do it properly and return Graham to his comrades and his family for burial. We also had to learn what we could. It became clear that the explosion had hurled his remains far and wide across a huge area of almost 75 by 200 metres. It was no wonder they couldn't find him at first. The closest piece was 60 metres away and the farthest 230 metres from the impact point.

We were able to show that his organs were all healthy, as you'd expect in a fit young fighter pilot. An oddity was he had an 11 per cent saturation with carbon monoxide. This seemed high, as we usually saw only four to five per cent in smokers and 55 to 60 per cent in carbon monoxide poisonings due to accident and suicide. There had been cases reported of pilots dying in-flight of carbon monoxide poisoning from faulty heaters in aircraft, but this level was far too low to cause any mental incapacitation. Eventually, although we had no definitive explanation, we decided it did not indicate an excessive or dangerous exposure. I believe FO Carter must have been unconscious after the impact with NZ 6211, because with his superb reflexes and training to expect the unexpected, he certainly had enough time — even if only just enough — to eject before striking the ground.

Flying Officer Graham Carter received a full military funeral, conducted in an Ohakea hangar amongst his beloved Skyhawks.

Flying Officer Graham Carter. 24 October 1989.
Requiescat in pace.

Ake Ake Kia Kaha.
For Ever and Ever be Strong
— Motto of 75 Squadron, Royal New Zealand Airforce

* * *

Not all fatal accidents are accidental, or necessarily even physical and causing traumatic injury.

Unfortunate Deaths

That may sound an odd thing to say, but what the coroner sometimes finds is that a death is 'accidental' only in the sense that it's not natural and the deceased didn't do it on purpose, as in a suicide. They simply made a fatal mistake.

So it was with one puzzle we had to unravel in Pahiatua. It began when we learned that a young man was dead in a home on the Mangaramarama Road in Tararua.

'Shae was with his mates, doing whatever mates do,' I explained to Kirsty, the very capable senior registrar tasked with investigating the case. 'He was last seen alive at 11 p.m. His mates found him on a couch at 2 a.m. and he couldn't be roused. They told the police that Shae suffered from asthma and he was on inhalers for this, although there weren't actually any inhalers in the house at that point. So mates hanging out into the wee hours, doing nothing and seeing nothing. Sounds improbable, doesn't it? What d'you think?'

Kirsty is bright and had seen this all before.

'Drugs?'

I nodded. It had to be drugs. I told Kirsty that I had heard an identical story in Levin in 1988. The patient back then was a 20-year-old lad named Darren Greco. He had apparently arrived at a friend's house, emotional but physically still okay. Then he was apparently struck with some kind of seizure and died.

'They were doing nothing unusual before this happened,' I told Kirsty. 'They were adamant about that.'

'Yeah, right!' Kirsty murmured.

I smiled.

'"He was upset and depressed," his mates told the police. "We think he's taken his own life." Maybe, I thought, but I didn't jump to any conclusions before I'd had a look. Turned out he had lethal levels of cocaine on board. As I said to the coroner, Graham Hubbard, no matter how you play this, common sense tells me they were all taking drugs big time at the party but he was the one to die from it. And they're covering it up.'

'Sounds similar,' Kirsty observed.

'Go find out,' I said. 'The answer surely must be there.'

Kirsty did a brilliant job. She found it, just as I knew she would. The autopsy and examination of Shae's body revealed nothing to give us a medical cause of death. As with my ancient case from Levin, toxicology had the answers. She brought the ESR lab report to me. I scanned through it and looked up at Kirsty in disbelief.

'Really? Clozapine?'

I was fully expecting methamphetamine, cocaine — anything but clozapine at therapeutic levels, no, never.

'That's not a drug of abuse, is it? I've never heard of it giving a high before.'

'I looked up its effects,' Kirsty answered. 'It's definitely not a drug of abuse. In fact, it's actually used to block highs and can be used to treat drug abusers.'

'So Shae's medical history must be wrong, surely? He must be a psychiatric patient to be on clozapine treatment. That's the only way I can think of that he'd get hold of it. If that's the case, his mates may not even have known about it, of course.'

'I've checked that out already.' Of course she had. 'I've checked with his GP and he doesn't know about him being on clozapine at all. There's no evidence anywhere that he's ever been on it.'

'So how'd it get in his blood?' I mused. That was the first

question to answer. The second was whether this level of the drug could actually kill him.

The second question was easier to answer than the first.

Yes, was the answer. Not a straightforward yes, but definitely a yes.

Clozapine has a number of effects on the heart, including occasionally sudden death in the vulnerable. This arises from an arrhythmia with the exotic name torsades de pointes. It sounds like a Spanish bullfight to me, which isn't far off the truth: like torsades de pointes, bullfights are invariably fatal, sometimes for the toreador, almost always for the bull.

'So where'd the clozapine come from? Who gave it to him? You don't just get it in your bloodstream like that!' I clicked my fingers.

A police team headed by Grayson Joines headed out grimly determined to find the answer. It was a protracted process but eventually one of the three lads who had been present at the death confessed. They had found the pills somewhere in a mate's cupboard and decided they were worth a try in the hopes they would cause a high. They took them even though they had no idea what they were — a kind of Russian roulette, as one of them described it to the coroner.

Shae died shortly after taking the pills.

His panicked mates burned the remaining pills and packaging in the fireplace and agreed not to talk to the police about it. For their part, the police were disappointed that their lack of honesty had contributed to a significant waste of time and effort, but the boys' actions weren't actually criminal.

I always feel sad at the death of a young person, and this hasn't diminished over the years despite seeing so many.

I suppose it's human nature to feel protective of the young. But it's far worse when the death is as needless as Shae's. How can you do such a stupid thing as take unknown pills you just found in a cupboard somewhere? It seems the young — and young men in particular — live in a golden haze of invincibility and no-one can tell them any different.

Shae Hemopo. 7 July 2012. Requiescat in pace.

* * *

Deaths for a good cause, while tragic, are somehow easier to bear. Sometimes we can even be uplifted by them.

It was early December 2016 and we were looking forward to Christmas. The rain had been very heavy but it was Thursday night and the weekend was at hand. There was only Friday to go, and work would soon be over for the week.

'The rain's holding off. I'd better get back and walk my dog along the river,' I remarked as my colleagues and I headed out to the car park.

'Bit wet down there, isn't it?'

'Not for her. She'll be into the river, given half a chance. See you tomorrow!'

It was very wet underfoot and my boots sank and sucked in the mud of the bridle path along the river bank. Scattered puddles of fresh rainwater washed them clean again and Tzinza, my golden Labrador bitch, galloped through the puddles in a shower of spray, her laughing face spotted with raindrops and her tongue lolling. We reached a beach formed where the first of a series of groynes — lines of solid steel posts marching down into the river — have been placed to deflect the Manawatu River in flood away from the expensive homes of Hokowhitu and the lower reaches of Palmerston North city.

Tzinza made to leap in and swim out to midstream as she had done practically every day for years, ever since she was a puppy. But not today. She hesitated.

She looked at the raging river for a long time, her twitching nose gathering information that is inaccessible to mere humans. And then, as I watched, she suddenly made a decision. She turned away from the river, chastened but determined.

She trotted back to my side and we turned for home.

My phone started beeping to register incoming text messages. Then it began to ring. Someone plainly wanted to talk to me. I answered.

'Are you all right?' It was Elayne. 'Thank God!'

'Why shouldn't I be? I'm just walking the dog.'

'A man walking his dog just where you are there has fallen in the river. Both he and his dog are gone. I thought it was you.'

I heard distant sirens wailing, drawing closer. The beat of helicopter rotors followed as darkness gathered over the raging river and the sodden soil.

Mike Toon was a highly respected police prosecutor. He was walking down the Manawatu that evening with his daughter and her dog. If all had gone as planned and Tzinza had taken her usual dip, they would have arrived on the scene within five minutes. But all did not go to plan.

Their beloved dog fell in the fast-flowing river and struggled to get back to the bank. Mike's daughter went to the rescue, and the angry river snatched her away, too. Mike reacted instinctively and dived in after her. He was a pretty good swimmer and, with his help, his daughter regained the bank. Their dog swam clear across the river and climbed ashore, unharmed, on the far side. But the river was terrible and implacable, running, as I later learned, at four times its usual volume. It took Mike Toon into its clutches and didn't let him go.

It was 9.30 a.m. on Friday, the following morning, when divers brought Mike away from the beach at that first groyne, the very spot where Tzinza's survival instinct had told her to stay out of the water. His body was carried from the river before an honour guard of his brother and sister officers.

Mike Toon died a good death for a good cause. In our sorrow, in our hearts, we knew that, and it was consolation for all of us. Mike was of that group of men of whom the Matabele would have said: 'They were men of men, and their fathers were men before them.'

Mike Toon. 1 December 2016. Requiescat in pace.

CHAPTER 11

We've Made a Dreadful Mistake

'We've made a dreadful mistake.' The young medical registrar wore his stethoscope draped around his neck like a badge of office. But he was clearly uneasy as he stood in my office. 'Can you do a post-mortem? The family are pretty unhappy with us.'

I could see he wasn't comfortable making eye contact. I was gentle with him.

'Tell me what happened.'

Mrs Eileen Anderson was 91 years of age and was in good health generally. She lived at Te Whanau Rest Home in Levin. She walked slowly with a stick or a frame but was mentally sharp and able to do her own cleaning and cooking.

'Eileen was brought to ED about midnight one night early this month. I saw her then. She was a bit deaf but fully conscious and mentally competent. She answered all my questions with no problems, if I asked them loudly enough.

She was really anxious about coming in but she settled fine after a cup of tea.'

It's fascinating how efficacious the humble cuppa is. Whether it's the comfort and warmth, the ritual familiarity or the ingredients within the brew itself probably doesn't matter. Tea is at the very core of our culture, and scientists have proven that it does in fact reduce stress. I drink tea all day and every day and it sure keeps me going.

'I admitted her because I thought she had a lung infection and so I started her on antibiotics. She wasn't actually given them at all that night because there was some mix-up on the ward and they couldn't find the right ones.'

I interrupted.

'Would you like a cup of tea?' I asked. 'I'm going to get one for myself.'

He nodded gratefully, but I saw he chose coffee from the cafeteria. The young doctors all do that these days. In some ways 'going out for a coffee' seems to have replaced the 'smoko' — the communal cigarette break — as a workplace social ritual.

Once we both had our hot drinks, I got him settled comfortably in a chair. I could see the story was going to be long and complicated. He relaxed visibly as he got into the flow of his tale.

'Dr Hayhurst is the consultant and he saw Eileen on the ward round the next morning.'

I knew Mike Hayhurst well from Africa. He had been a medical registrar specialising in respiratory medicine when I was a pathology registrar back in Cape Town in the early 1980s. He was a very good physician.

'He heard crepitations at the base of the left lung and

diagnosed pneumonia, even though there were no changes yet in her chest X-ray. We started her on roxithromycin. I charted it on her medication chart, which was with her notes.'

I thought I detected a quaver in his voice. He paused, and swallowed.

'She was feeling better and her blood oxygen saturation was fine so we decided to send her home. That took most of the day to get organised but her discharge summary was typed up and she was ready to go by late evening. I hadn't seen her again after the ward round but she was up and mobilising well that morning. After lunch she suddenly became quite drowsy and lethargic. By that evening she was confused, too. The nursing staff didn't like the look of things and sent for the Med B registrar on call to examine her. Her discharge was cancelled. She slept soundly all night and was more alert and not confused by morning. Again it was decided to discharge her.'

He shook his head.

'But it happened again. By evening she was confused and disorientated and unable to feed herself. Her daughter was really concerned at her decline in hospital over the two days since Saturday. We just didn't get what was happening. We missed it completely.'

I knew the crunch was coming.

'What happened?' I asked gently.

'It wasn't *her* medication chart that I wrote on that was filed in her notes. She was given another patient's medications.'

'Oh God, no!' I couldn't help myself. 'What was she given?'

'The worst was morphine sulphate.'

'Morphine! How much? I mean, what dose?'

'One hundred milligrams, twice a day.'

'*What?* That's 20 times the usual dose! Who in hell is on that?'

'There's another patient with long-standing chronic pain. They've been on it for a while and have become tolerant so they need a much higher dose. It's that other patient's chart that got mixed up in Eileen's notes.'

I was stunned. That was a massive dose of morphine. No wonder she became sleepy and confused. By rights it should have killed her outright.

'You said morphine was the worst. Were there other drugs, too?'

He nodded. 'Quite a few. Warfarin, isosorbide, Losec and oxybutynin were also on the chart with the morphine. None of them were her meds but she got them all.'

'Hmm. Not good, but they shouldn't pose too much of a problem with toxicity. I suppose they were all at usual doses? No other surprises like the morphine?'

'No, they were okay.'

'So what happened to her? The morphine would cause a profound respiratory depression, wouldn't it?'

'It took us a couple of days to twig. She lived a further two weeks after we discovered the mistake and put her on her correct treatment. But it knocked her back quite a bit and she never really got back to her condition on admission. After that, Eileen was often confused even though the morphine was gone from her system and she wasn't really able to look out for herself. Her pneumonia wouldn't clear up and, in fact, we thought it was getting worse. She went into heart and renal failure and died just after breakfast yesterday.'

'Oh dear. That's just terrible. I presume you've informed the police and the coroner?'

'Yes. The coroner wants a post-mortem.'

* * *

Eileen was a gentle-looking, frail lady. I saw she had an old mastectomy scar and read that the procedure had been carried out back in 1954. My God, that was the year I was born! It made me feel suddenly very old.

There was some varicose eczema and a clean heel ulcer, both common amongst those in their tenth decade of life. More ominous was the swelling of the legs, signalling heart failure.

It was pointless sending blood for toxicology now, but I did it anyway, more in the event a court case arose than with any expectation of finding morphine. After two weeks, all traces of the morphine and other drugs would have long since been purged from her body and, indeed, her blood tests were negative.

The cause of death was to be found in her lungs, of course. They were both very heavy and solid, weighing in at just under a kilogram each. That's mighty heavy for a little lady whose usual lung weight sits at about a third of that. They both looked about as badly diseased as each other, even though the doctors had thought that the main site of the pneumonia was the left lung.

I gently squeezed the lungs and clear fluid poured out.

'That's pulmonary oedema. I am sure that developed from her heart failure. Heart failure must have been her final event.'

I selected blocks of tissue from each of the lung lobes to examine under the microscope and to prove the diagnosis of pneumonia.

I was surprised at what I saw. It wasn't the solid plugging of the alveoli — the air sacs — with inflammatory white cells that I had expected to see in a classical, bacterial pneumonia. It had gone way past that early consolidation stage. Scarring had now blossomed in the air sacs and it had become an organising pneumonia.

'That's what happens when pneumonia fails to get better,' I explained to my young registrar, who was seeing what I was seeing on my double-header microscope. 'The body gives up and just scars and blocks up the air sacs, a bit like pouring a barrow of cement down your kitchen sink when you can't unblock it. It's a bad development and it doesn't get better. The lungs start failing to deliver oxygen. But look at this. There's more. See these pink membranes lining the surfaces of many of the air sacs? Those are hyaline membranes from fibrin leaking out from her bloodstream. They are a sign of what we call diffuse alveolar damage, or DAD.'

'What does it mean in her case?'

'Good question. It used to be called Vietnam lung, or sometimes shock lung. It was discovered back in the Vietnam War when soldiers were unlucky enough to have their mouths open when mortar rounds burst near them. They took the full shock of the blast right in their lungs. They were then usually also pumped full of saline fluid by enthusiastic medics who knew no better. The lungs were overloaded from the transfusions and shocked by the blast and so threw in the towel and just tried to wall themselves off from the world. That's what those pink membranes are doing. They're drawing the curtains closed on an unfixable injury.'

Shock lung wasn't confined to the battlefield, I explained. For once it had been recognised, we found it to be relatively common even in civilian patients.

'We now call it ARDS, or adult respiratory distress syndrome. We see it everywhere in our hospitals, now. There are heaps of other causes. In Eileen's case, it could be anything from bacteria and viruses to the industrial doses of morphine, which would have had the effect of stopping her coughing and perhaps even caused her to inhale some of her stomach acids while unconscious. Hydrochloric acid is pretty savagely destructive and dissolves the tissues when you suck it into the lung. Her age, too, would be a bit against her in any pneumonia, even without the morphine.'

I knew the timing of the changes we were looking at would be an important question, especially if the morphine was to be implicated.

'The ARDS has been here several days at least. The organising pneumonia pre-dates it. I would put this level of fibrous organisation and scarring at two to three weeks.'

There was no doubt in my mind. That sat pretty much squarely around the time of her first admission.

Mike Hayhurst told me later: 'We just missed it. We would see her on ward rounds day after day and sometimes she would be pretty good, and then out of nowhere she would suddenly deteriorate again. Of course, now it's blindingly obvious that Eileen went downhill after lunch each day shortly after she was topped up with the next mega-dose of morphine. The penny just didn't drop. It's not something you expect to see in a hospital, though. You just don't even consider it as a remote possibility.'

* * *

We were called to the Coroners Court for an inquest. This would be a bigger affair than usual. There were to be lawyers from the hospital, lawyers from the family, family members up from Levin and, no doubt, the press, too. Serious and weighty questions were certainly going to be asked. I couldn't advise the hospital's lawyers beforehand as I was the advisor to the coroner, but my colleagues had been consulted by them and had given their views.

We always met in the District Court for coronial hearings but that morning the police phoned to tell me of a change of venue.

'It's been transferred to the Kingsgate Hotel.'

'The Kingsgate? Why?'

'We don't know. Graham Hubbard told us to move it there only last night. I think he doesn't want the press there and this might throw them off the scent.'

It was possible, I suppose. Graham hated publicity. He was always jovial and friendly in court but I had once seen him tear strips off a reporter who annoyed him.

Anyway, we duly convened in the conference centre at the hotel at 10 a.m. sharp. Besides me, there were the family, the lawyers, Mike Hayhurst and Catherine Jackson, the hospital radiologist. The press were nowhere in sight.

'All rise for the coroner,' a policeman called out.

'Be seated. I see there are no reporters here today?' Graham pleasantly addressed the policeman.

'No sir. They weren't informed of the change of venue.'

'I must apologise for that oversight on my part,' he said, beaming at us all. 'Shall we begin, then?'

The story was exactly as I had heard it and it was all quite uncontroversial. Mike indicated that as the consultant in charge, he accepted full responsibility and he explained the dangerous existing system of charting patients' medication that led to the error had not been recognised. As a matter of routine, Catherine Jackson finished describing the changes in the chest X-ray to the court. But then the hospital's lawyer rose to question her.

'Surely the lung changes show the pneumonia is not all that important? After all, you've just told us it is a small pneumonia. That wouldn't kill her, surely?'

Everyone present recognised this as a possible attempt to try to minimise the hospital's culpability. The lawyer doubtless felt it was his duty to the hospital, but it was ill-considered.

'I never said it was small,' Catherine snapped. 'I said the X-ray appearances were subtle. That's quite a different thing.'

It wasn't a helpful question really and would have proved nothing. It was an example of the worst aspect of our adversarial system. The autopsy had already shown massive, widespread damage, and Eileen had died from it. You couldn't get more serious than that. There wasn't much more to add, really. We had made a fatal mistake and Eileen died from it.

The hearing continued on to its predictable conclusion, and in a technical and legal sense, this tragic episode was at a close. But I'm sure it never ended for the family, who must have been left wondering why it had to happen. It would be hard for them to trust the medical system as fully as they had before. After all, people take their life, their most precious asset, and put it trustingly into our hands. What are they to think when we drop it so clumsily?

I know it profoundly affected the doctors and nurses involved, too. Mike and I spoke of Eileen many times afterwards and before his own sad and early death. He used to shake his head and say: 'We just never even thought that accidental doses of morphine was a possibility.'

Yet it had happened before and it will certainly happen again. Medication mistakes are common in hospitals around the world, apparently affecting one in six patients; most mistakes don't result in harm, but about one in a hundred causes an injury. Eileen's case was at the more extreme end.

I have personal experience of how easily it can happen.

When my youngest daughter, Charlotte, was eight months old, she developed childhood cancer, a yolk sac tumour. She was admitted to Wellington Hospital for chemotherapy and Elayne went along to care for her. One morning, the oncology staff came to hang the bag containing her daily dose of cisplantin from the infusion stand. As a haematologist, Elayne was very familiar with the protocols and the use of these toxic drugs and she spotted that the wrong dose had been calculated. Charlotte would have been given ten times her correct dose if Elayne had not been there.

We are not robots. Medical professionals are all human, and so long as that's the case, we'll surely make errors in whatever we do.

Eileen Maud Anderson. 22 April 2002. Requiescat in pace.

We've Made a Dreadful Mistake

* * *

Diagnosis in medicine is often difficult. At least, it is using the human brain, which is all that most doctors have at their disposal. Maybe artificial intelligence will see advances made in this frustrating task: Dr Google is frequently consulted by patients and is surprisingly good. Patients often present knowing more than their doctors about their symptoms from their internet searches. That is perhaps a harbinger of a brighter future for medicine.

Diagnosis is particularly difficult in the Emergency Department, which is constantly, endlessly besieged by hundreds of patients. 'Patient' is an apt word, for that is what you have to be: very, very patient. Waiting times can be hours, sometimes up to six or even more. The smaller centres like Masterton and Gisborne smoke it, but the bigger you get, it seems, the longer the wait. Palmerston North has an ED of just the right size to become a bastard. If you have to visit our Emergency Department, you will wait.

The problem confronting us and Emergency Departments everywhere is that there is a mix of patients. Some don't have a lot wrong with them, or nothing a GP couldn't fix. But their GP charges 30, 40 or even 50 dollars for a consultation, whereas the Emergency Department is free. For many, a five- or six-hour wait is a fair exchange for fifty bucks saved. This inevitably means ED waiting rooms are stuffed full of people who should be seeing their GP but who can't really afford to, rubbing shoulders with genuine emergency cases — the injured and the truly sick, who really need attention. Trouble is, you can't tell at a glance who is who, and the triage process — sorting them into categories of need —

can be time-consuming and a real drain on resources. We used to say in Africa that you have to sift a lot of dirt to find a nugget of gold. And it is equally true that you have to sift through a heap of patients to find the one desperately deserving of your time and care. You don't have much time to listen and to look and to palpate and to diagnose. It's a difficult speciality and the ED doctors are really good at it. There just aren't enough of them.

The health bureaucrats have the answer. Of course they do. They just made a rule to control it.

In New Zealand, they decreed, 90 per cent of ED patients will be seen within six hours. In the National Health Service in the United Kingdom, it is only four hours. That'll fix it, the bureaucrats have decided. On the 'how', they are silent, and the rule has created some strange and undesirable outcomes. In England, ED doctors have told me they sometimes see patients outside in the ambulances and keep them there until they can admit them directly to a ward. Time in an ambulance isn't logged and doesn't count towards the four-hour limit, you see. This way, they don't stuff up the bureaucrats' statistics, which keeps everyone happy — apart, of course, from the patients.

* * *

My office phone jangled early one morning. I was surprised. Who was this phoning my office at such an unsocial hour? It was only 7.30 a.m. I was already at work because I had a big backlog of cases and had come in for an early start. But no-one knew I was there. I should have had an uninterrupted hour to catch up.

'Good morning, Doc. Glad we found you in. We phoned you at home and your wife gave us this number.'

It was the Palmerston North police station, which was odd. Not the CIB: we're used to calls from them at all hours, which invariably means serious work is afoot. The local station was where they locked up drunks and petty crooks caught going about their nefarious business.

'We've got a curly one here we need help on. It's a death in custody.'

I was puzzled.

'Don't deaths in custody have to be referred to the coroner? I thought that was the law.'

'Yep, that's right. But he's not in actual custody, you see.'

'So what's the problem?'

'Well, one of our patrol cars was on State Highway 57 out towards Linton Army Camp late last night and they spotted a man walking along the road. About halfway between here and the camp. But he didn't seem quite right.'

Halfway would be about eight kilometres out over the other side of the bridge over the Manawatu River. Pretty much the middle of nowhere.

'What do you mean "not right"?'

'Sort of just shambling along. Like going nowhere. But they recognised him straight away. It was Jazz Moffitt. We know him.'

'Why? Has he got a record?'

Was this going to be another paedophile story or a gang-related death, or was it something worse?

'No, not Jazz. He's just a bit of a layabout. Hangs around the fringes of petty crime a bit. He's homeless, mainly hanging around the Levin area. No fixed address. We quite like him.'

'So how has he come to be dead and not in custody, then?'

The officers had braked, pulled over and got out to talk to Jazz.

'Where're you off to at this time of night, Jazz?'

'To Levin. I'm headed back there.'

'It's 11 o'clock, mate, and that's 40 kilometres away. You won't get there till tomorrow. What're you doing here in Palmy?'

'I'm pretty crook. Guts ache and sick. Came up to the ED to see someone here in Palmy. Nobody was interested in me in Levin.'

'So what happened?'

'Waited all afternoon there in ED before the doctor saw me. Said there was nothing wrong with me and discharged me.'

He looked at the cops, a scrawny, grubby and pallid face, not exactly in the pink of health.

'Told me I could go home, like it was some sort of treat for me. Got no home and got no money here, so I'm walking back to Levin.'

Which was, as the police had pointed out, still an eight-hour walk away. The police officers maybe saw some mother's vulnerable child there. They knew there wasn't a bad bone in Jazz's body.

'Get in the car, mate. You can sleep in the station tonight and we'll get you back to Levin tomorrow.'

I was impatient to get to the important part of the story. The death.

'And?'

'We brought him back here to the station and put him up in a cell. One of the men went out to the BP station and bought him a pie because he hadn't eaten all day. It was the only place that was open.'

I bet it was their own money they used to buy the pie. I wasn't sure they were even allowed to put people up in the cells like that. I suspected not. But that's what the police do.

'What sort of pie was it?' I asked.

'Just a chicken pie.'

'And now he's dead?'

'Yes.' The officer didn't sound at all happy.

'Not surprised,' I said. 'Chicken pies especially can be lethal.'

I was pulling his leg, of course. Chicken pies are fine. Mostly.

* * *

The old Palmerston North police lock-up looked ancient to me: not Dickensian, not quite Victorian, but not too modern, either. It was maybe built in the 1950s, with thick, cold concrete walls — newly painted, but still blank and grim — steel bars to break your spirit and thick doors which were distinctly metallic and heavy. But for Jazz, who lay on a bench-like bed recessed into the wall, those doors were wide open. He could have walked out anytime he wanted.

He wasn't in custody, but it only took a few seconds' examination to establish that he was most certainly dead.

'He looks pretty crook,' observed the sergeant.

'Pretty dead, too. So yes, you're right. Pretty damn crook,' I replied, although I know what he meant. Some people manage to look robustly healthy even when they're dead, sometimes better than when they were alive. But poor old

Jazz was white, drawn and haggard, his pallor accentuated by his grey stubble. His mouth hung open in an unbecoming O, as if sucking thick air into reluctant lungs.

He looked sick. I was sure as anything that he was, and that there was medical mischief to be found within.

'Let's get him up to the mortuary and see what your chicken pie has done,' I said. I was trying to be light-hearted to lift their anxiety. It didn't really work. Deaths in custody are taken very, very seriously. They all have to be reported to the coroner, we have to autopsy them and there has to be an investigation.

'But we got the pie from the local petrol station,' the sergeant protested anxiously. 'We eat them ourselves, all the time.'

'Don't worry, mate, I'm just taking the piss. It'll be okay.'

The autopsy was indeed okay, at least from the perspective of the police and their potentially dodgy pie.

We split the chest cavity and plucked the lungs and heart out in a block. I nicked a hole in the pericardium and slit the membrane open, peeling it back to reveal the heart. There it lay in its perfection, glistening like a tropical mango, sweet and perfect. I flicked it over to look at the back.

'Oh, fuck!' I said involuntarily, mentally apologising to my gentle mum and mother-in-law, who wouldn't have approved of this kind of language. 'Look at this!'

The back of the heart was bruised and blue over a vast area. This was a massive heart attack, a posterior wall infarct.

We all know about heart attacks. In these well-informed, well-equipped times, there's a whole cohort of society who keep tabs on where the closest defibrillator is, and who're always half on the lookout for a middle-aged white male falling to his knee, clutching his chest and complaining of crushing chest pain radiating to his left shoulder.

Trouble is, not all heart attacks are quite like that. I recall a story from Africa of a middle-aged executive playing a golf ball from the rough, coming out holding his head in his hands and collapsing unresponsive to the ground. Heart attacks on golf courses are not uncommon and there are plans and facilities to deal with this — not to mention higher than usual concentrations of medically qualified personnel on hand, given the game's popularity amongst the medical profession. Sophisticated resuscitation was therefore close at hand. But in this particular instance, the efforts of all concerned didn't work out.

It turned out there was quite a big black mamba living in the tree under which his ball had landed. And the snake hit him a glancing shot on his scalp just behind his ear. He possibly never even realised what had happened. Not that it would have made any difference if he had, not with a mamba. Their neurotoxin is fast, very fast, and can easily mimic a sudden heart attack. In fact, the death does result from a sort of heart attack, I suppose.

But some genuine heart attacks can kill just as insidiously as a mamba and are particularly hard to diagnose. I have seen many of these in both the quick and the dead: like Jazz, they often complain of a guts ache and feel a little bit crook. It's not very dramatic, but it can be suddenly and unexpectedly fatal. Sometimes their symptoms are so minor that the family just can't accept the diagnosis.

I remember another patient of mine, who had died from just such a heart attack, being the subject of an inquest before Graham Hubbard. It was a difficult inquest, because the family were angry about everything.

'We took him twice to the doctor, paid both times. He told us it was only guts ache. He said it was probably gastritis or gallstones or something, but the waiting list at the hospital for an X-ray was nine months.'

I could see quite clearly what the cause of their anger was, as I listened to them that day in the Coroners Court. People trust doctors to get it right, but what if we don't? Could we have done better for their father and husband? It's possible, but the odds are against it, I'm afraid. We're amazingly good at parts of the game of life, disease and death. We're just not that good at the diagnostic part of the game, especially early in the story when the signs and symptoms are subtle and we really have to use our brains.

Graham Hubbard knew this for he was a wise coroner. He always told the truth but I think he sometimes chose to speak in parables, just as Our Lord did so long ago.

'Well,' he said sympathetically, leaning forward over the bench, 'your practitioner has rightly told you that your husband and father had gastritis. Now as I understand it, "gastritis" is a very non-specific term indicating something beneath is seriously amiss. It's more of a description of symptoms, not a diagnosis as such.'

Graham was blessed with the face of a grandfather everyone loves and trusts. He smiled benevolently on the family, and in the face of his combined magisterial mana and his evident compassion, all the anger went out of them.

Graham Hubbard may not even have been quite correct about the difference between gastritis and a heart attack, but he knew people and how to soothe their emotions. Sometimes that skill is even better than being factually correct and technically perfect. It was enough that day.

We've Made a Dreadful Mistake

So Jazz had suffered a massive heart attack, of this insidious, silent type. He had felt bad, of course, bad enough to seek medical help. But his heart attack was just a bit too silent to be obvious.

'It wasn't your BP chicken pie, after all. This lets you folk off, for sure. It was a straightforward heart attack.'

The police officers breathed a sigh of relief.

But I had a duty to perform with the Emergency Department doctors. If the dead do not teach the living, how will we ever learn? I went to tell them Jazz's story.

'So, that's it. There was a right coronary artery thrombus, a posterior wall infarct about four to five days old. That was the final diagnosis.'

I was drinking unpleasantly strong coffee in the ED consultant's office. I suppose they need weapons-grade coffee to keep them going through the long hours between the middle of the night and dawn.

'A difficult diagnosis,' he grimaced, staring at Jazz's ED notes. 'Not sure I can add anything else, now. We thought it was maybe a minor gastric upset and he was okay to go. We didn't know about him being homeless and walking back to Levin. What a stuff-up. I guess we just made a dreadful mistake here, didn't we?'

He shook his head sadly. Emergency Department doctors have a weight of sorrows to bear that equal — might even surpass — the weight we bear in the mortuary.

'Jazz' Moffitt. July 1989. Requiescat in pace.

* * *

The Quick and the Dead

No-one told me when I became a doctor how depressingly common mistakes are in medicine. It is a lesson I have learned down the years. Some, as above, are mistakes of diagnosis, some of treatment, some arise where the wrong medicine or the wrong dose is accidentally administered. And some are a wholesale failure of knowledge and application and resources. I spent part of my years as a young doctor administering completely the wrong treatment to patients, because medicine itself simply had the theory of the disease woefully wrong.

Let me give you an example.

My patient was a computer analyst called Hans Voteller, young and with the patchy sort of beard made popular by Yasser Arafat. I saw him in Casualty, which is what we used to call the Emergency Department. He was pale and anxious-looking. He had vomited blood twice that night. I put a drip up and started running in saline while I waited for units of blood to be cross-matched.

I paged Mr Gerry Divaris, the general surgeon in charge, to examine him. I outlined Hans's history.

'He has a high-stress job, eats irregularly and smokes 60 cigarettes a day. He says he's had indigestion for several months. He reckons it's his irregular hours.'

Mr Divaris nodded. 'What's his haemoglobin?'

'Eight grams. His blood pressure and pulse are all right, though.'

'Must be a bleeder. Probably a DU. Get him up to theatre and I'll 'scope him and see what's up. Please arrange that and call me when it's ready.'

I explained this to Hans. 'We think you may have a duodenal ulcer which is bleeding. Mr Divaris is going to pass a gastroscope into your stomach and have a look.'

We've Made a Dreadful Mistake

He nodded his agreement. 'All right, Doctor. Will I need an operation?'

'Possibly, although bleeding ulcers often settle by themselves. We'll know more once we've had a look. Then we'll decide what the next move is.'

'We're in the duodenum. Have a look.' Mr Divaris beckoned me over to look into the eyepiece of the gastroscope. 'There it is.'

I could see the ugly crater of an ulcer on the mucosa, and as I watched, it filled with blood with each heartbeat, gushing like a geyser.

'It's on the posterior wall of the duodenum,' he explained to me. 'The artery is eroded and is too large to seal itself. The blood will pump out as fast as we can put it in. I'll have to open him up.'

As the house surgeon, it was my job to explain everything to Hans, arrange the anaesthetist and spar with the theatre matron for an urgent operating theatre. And all the while, I also had to manage Hans's blood and fluids to keep him stable until I handed him over to the anaesthetist. Then I had to scrub to assist Mr Divaris during the surgery. Afterwards, I would have to get Hans back to the ward and supervise his post-operative care through the night. Back in the 1970s, working in a surgical firm was pretty tough.

Mr Divaris's knife expertly slit the skin and fat down to the fascia. A dozen capillaries flared, throwing up a fine red mist. Mr Divaris rapidly clipped them off with fine forceps.

'Diathermy.'

The instrument was passed to him. Each forceps was touched, and with a smoky flash, each bleeding vessel was cauterised closed. He split open the tendon of the abdominal wall and opened the delicate peritoneal membrane covering the intestines.

'Warm towel, please, sister.'

Heavy cloths soaked in saline were placed over the bowels which were pulled gently to the side.

'It's your job to hold everything out of the way, Cynric. And don't be rough. I don't want him getting an ileus.'

He deftly exposed the stomach and duodenum. The duodenal cap was swollen and scarred from the ulcer within. He packed towels around to mop up any spillage and slit the lower stomach and duodenum open. I could see the fresh blood welling out from the exposed ulcer. It swiftly and richly coloured the towels.

'Suture.' He held out his hand and the needle and catgut were immediately and expertly placed in it. With practised flicks of the curved needle, he sutured the ulcer base and tied a knot with one hand, sheathed as it was deep inside the abdomen.

The ulcer suddenly became bloodless as the artery was tied off.

So far this was great. This had saved Hans's life.

'Is everything all right to carry on?' Mr Divaris looked at the anaesthetist, who nodded.

He closed the slit between the stomach and duodenum in such a way as to open widely the passage from the stomach into the duodenum. 'That's a pyloroplasty to create drainage,' he explained briefly to me. I knew that. I had studied all these procedures for my final exams only the previous year.

He then proceeded to dissect the great vagus nerve off the front of the stomach. Once he had located it, he cut it. Then he did the same on the back wall of the stomach. Apart from closing up, the operation was over, so he was rather more forthcoming.

'The vagus nerve supplies the acid-producing part of the stomach. Cut it and you can reduce the acid to nothing. Then the duodenal ulcer can heal.'

For such was the state of knowledge at the time. The first part of the operation to tie off the bleeder was lifesaving, but the second part, the severing of the vagus nerve, was a serious mistake. This was only one operation of thousands of identical ones done in hospitals all around the developed world, every single day.

You see, at the time, peptic ulcer disease was almost an epidemic in the West and it was getting worse. We knew exactly what caused it. It was our stomach pouring too much acid into the duodenum, the section of gut into which it empties. The excess acid dissolved the very lining of the gut. And what caused the stomach to do this destructive thing? We knew that for certain, too, because they told us in our lectures with all the authority that modern medical wisdom could muster. It was the chronic stress of our modern lives, and smoking and spicy foods, that had created this deadly acid tide.

We learned all about not only the vagotomy and drainage surgery such as Hans underwent, but also of Billroth I and Billroth II resections and complicated bypasses. Our surgical lists were packed with operations for peptic ulcer disease — and not a few others to correct the complications of previous ulcer surgery. One of the worst complications was 'dumping'. Because we enlarged the opening from the stomach, the undigested food would pass from the stomach directly into the small bowel, and it was too much, too rich and far too concentrated. The sufferer would get a feeling of fullness, pain, nausea, vomiting, flushing and diarrhoea. This occurred with every meal. Imagine how ghastly life must be with that to look forward to every single day. It's quite enough to put you right off your food for life.

And meanwhile, in cases not deemed serious enough for surgical intervention, we prescribed a welter of antacid potions and wrecked people's enjoyment of life by enforcing bland diets of milk and lightly poached white fish to staunch the acid flow.

Stress and spices, we thought. Caffeine and coffee. We were profoundly wrong in almost every case. Smoking and spirits did play a trivial role. But peptic ulcer disease is an infection. It is due to a bacterial organism. It never was fundamentally a surgical disease needing surgery in the first place. All it needed was simple antibiotics.

As early as 1958, a humble Greek general practitioner, John Lykoudis, thought so and treated his patients with antibiotics. He successfully treated more than thirty thousand patients with a cocktail of antibiotics that he had personally devised. Far from taking notice of his results, the Greek medical establishment punished him, effectively for heresy, much as the Catholic Church punished Galileo for being bold enough to speak the truth about the Earth orbiting the sun. Lykoudis was fined 4000 drachmas by a disciplinary committee and indicted in court. The *Journal of the American Medical Association* refused to publish his findings, to their eternal shame. As a result, three decades' worth of pointless and often debilitating surgery was performed on thousands of patients before Barry Marshall and Robin Warren in Perth, Australia, finally isolated *Helicobacter pylori* from the stomach in 1982. These bugs were the cause of the whole shemozzle. Marshall and Warren weren't entirely believed at first, either. To prove his point, Barry Marshall took the extreme measure of experimenting on himself. He drank a culture of the bacterium. Sure enough, he got the symptoms and they disappeared on antibiotics.

Acceptance was then swift. Antibiotics were given and the incidence of peptic ulcer disease dropped impressively. Surgical intervention was quietly shelved without so much as an embarrassed apology, and daily surgical lists were filled by patients in genuine need. Marshall and Warren were awarded the Nobel Prize for Physiology or Medicine in 2005. Dr John Lykoudis was never acknowledged, and is officially remembered only for his 'disgraceful' conduct.

Errare, as they say, *est humanum*: it is human to make mistakes. Fortunately, I don't know of another example of how the medical profession has systematically got something quite so wrong. I am sorry for my part in every misguided peptic ulcer disease procedure in which I was involved during those years. Yet I have to say that I still feel good about Hans Voteller, for he lived where he would certainly have died from blood loss, regardless of the misunderstanding of the underlying cause of his disease. I used to see him here and there about town over subsequent years and he looked fine. Once I met him at the local swimming pool and he showed me, and I admired, his healed scar. I gather he gave up smoking, which was one good outcome. I think — at least, I hope — he didn't suffer any of those ghastly complications from the unnecessary part of his surgery that we did that day, and I hope he has continued to enjoy a long and happy life.

CHAPTER 12

Perils in the Bush

The holiday week over the New Year period had been great, really hot and dry. Temperatures had soared to 28 degrees early in the week and stayed there. That made up for a cold, wet and very changeable December. At last families could get out under their poolside umbrellas, onto the beach or down by the river. So for most families, January 2003 was a time for enjoying life.

But not for all.

Jason Chase had been missing for three weeks, ever since 13 December. He was a 25-year-old shearer who had been staying up Tairawhiti way. He was fit and healthy with no known illnesses: in fact, he was in great shape, because he was training for a bike race. We knew he had left Gisborne back in mid-December and was headed back home to Dannevirke to his family for Christmas.

He never arrived.

At first this went unnoticed, as there wasn't a specific date for his arrival. Then an abandoned car was reported in the

Tamaki Reserve, just out of Dannevirke in the foothills of the Ruahine Range. It was Jason's car.

Why was it there? Where was Jason? What was he doing?

No-one knew. We heard he knew the area pretty well and he could easily have gone up into the mountains for a bit. But it was all really out of character. He had been somewhat depressed but there was nothing to suggest he was suicidal.

The search ground into gear.

The Palmerston North rescue helicopter flew several missions, weaving in and out of the steep-sided gullies so close that it seemed you could lean out and touch them as they passed. Eyes diligently scoured the ground beneath for any trace. What the searchers hope for is the lost soul to hear you and see you, and come out into sight waving. All efforts were fruitless. The search was officially suspended just before Christmas.

The festive season was a pretty bleak time for the Chase family. They weren't satisfied and understandably so. Jason's whanau and the Dannevirke community would not give up. Hundreds of volunteers rallied and continued their private search. They just knew he was up there.

Teams of rescuers went out each day to quarter large tracts of the mountains. It is a beautiful but wild place to tramp. If you get lost, it's a very hard place in which to be found. It's punishing terrain — very steep mountainsides clad in dense native bush with intervening, rock-strewn gullies. These gullies carry torrents of water in the wet season, but they were dry and hard and irregular going to walk along right now. Periodically, slips scar the steep sides of the ranges, disgorging yet more rocks into the gullies. In winter, as I look out of my office window, I can see the surrounding peaks are often dusted with snow.

The Quick and the Dead

The search went on day after day. A Pongaroa farmer even helped out using his aeroplane to see if he could find Jason.

But the search was a failure. There was no sign that Jason had even passed by anywhere there. If it weren't for the presence of his car, there would have been no reason to suppose he was in there at all.

Finally, around the middle of the afternoon on Friday, 3 January, I received a call.

'Sergeant Fincham, Dannevirke Police, Doctor. We've found Jason Chase.'

'Where was he? In the Ruahines?'

'Yep, he was up in the ranges okay and pretty much where we were searching.'

'How'd you find him?'

'We didn't. The whanau did. They've carried on searching up there ever since the official search was called off. Two of them found him just after midday today.'

'I'm assuming he's dead, since you're calling me. Does it look suspicious?'

'Yep, he's dead and has been for a while, I'd say. But it doesn't look suspicious, really. He's lying in a dry, rocky river bed right next to a small pool of water. We think he may have fallen but the men who found him reckon there's nowhere nearby that he could have fallen from. Maybe he fell somewhere else and staggered there with injuries.'

'Maybe. I'll need to see the scene or at least have good photographs so I can see the background context before I start the autopsy.'

'We've photographed everything and have also flown in a helicopter to get an aerial view.'

That was excellent news. The police had outdone themselves

getting all this done so quickly. I really didn't feel like a long slog up into the ranges this late on a Friday. The weather was really hot. It would have been hard yakka.

'There's another thing, Doc. The coroner, Mr Stuart Smith, has asked if you could do the autopsy urgently. Like, tonight.'

It was already late in the day. It would keep us there quite late at night. That was unusual.

'Yes, of course I can do it tonight. But what's the hurry? He's been dead a while so tomorrow morning isn't going to make so much difference, is it?'

'The family are really angry about all this. They reckon we stuffed up finding him back in December. Some say he was still alive and we just gave up too quickly. So we really need to know whether he'd been injured and how long he's been dead.'

'Okay. I'll do it tonight.'

'Oh, and one other thing. There are some maggots on the body. Can you collect them so we can see how long they've been around to date his death?'

'I'll do that. Although I thought that ideally you're supposed to do that first-up? You collect them at the scene from the body and the surroundings, don't you?'

'Oh.' He sounded disappointed. 'We didn't know that. We've already brought him out.'

'No worries. I'll do what I can. Can you bring Jason to the mortuary for us by six this evening?'

* * *

That evening, the police handed me a booklet of the beautifully taken pictures their photographer had prepared. I studied the photographs carefully, sitting dressed for action in my surgical scrubs in the tiny cupboard that served as the mortuary office.

The backdrop was typical Ruahine ranges and I was right about the temperature that day, as it was clearly baking in the sunshine. There was nothing visible in the gully from 500 feet, but as the photographer descended, there, quite clearly, was Jason.

He was easy to see, as he was wearing a short-sleeved, multi-coloured rugby shirt with a bright-red back displayed to the sky. His pale shorts were either cream-coloured or were a very faded khaki. He was lying peacefully on his left side with his legs stretched out and his feet bare. If he hadn't been on a rocky river bed, you'd have thought he'd just lain down there for a comfortable snooze.

The police were right. This was certainly no murder scene. It looked peaceful. There had been no deadly struggle here, and I was sure he had died exactly on this spot. I could easily imagine him lying down here for the last time, making himself as comfortable as he could.

'Right, gentlemen. Should we start?'

The CIB investigation team was there and ready to go. They were treating this death very seriously. As usual, Steve was the scene of crime officer, in charge of collecting and collating all the bits of evidence. He produced an insect field collection kit. This was the first official one I'd ever seen and I had no idea of what to do with it. I was interested to see what results it would yield.

'Can you collect the insects?' he said, grinning. I think he could see I was quite at sea, staring at the insect life seething from the unzipped body bag.

'I'll try.'

I collected ten sample pots in the end. I plucked the maggots one by one — from Jason himself, of course: from his eye sockets, chest, back and hands. There were lots inside the body bag where they had fallen off, so I scooped up a few pots of those, too. Most looked the same to my untrained eye but there were a few that were a little different, so I added them to the mix.

I thought I had read somewhere that you're supposed to kill the animals as soon as you collect them, so as to prevent them advancing in their developmental cycle and confusing the chronology.

'There you go. Top them up with 100 per cent alcohol to kill them.'

I handed the pots over to Steve with a shudder of revulsion. There's something downright disgusting about wriggling maggots. I can't stomach them.

I examined Jason carefully from head to toe. He had no injuries at all. His skin was blistered here and there from the onset of putrefaction, but only on his lower legs and arms. The biggest blister was ten centimetres across, but most were tiny. There was no greenish-black marbling of the veins over his abdominal skin and no greening of the skin over his colon.

This certainly wasn't impressive or advanced decay.

The tissue within his chest lying between his heart and lungs felt like bubble wrap, crackling and popping as I rubbed it between my fingers.

'Crepitus,' I murmured aloud to myself.

'Crap—? What crap is that, Doc?' A constable was standing behind me, a biro poised over his notepad.

I smiled. 'No. Not crap. Crepitus. It's these bubbles. They're from gas-forming bugs and are a sign of decay. This is still early. Later the gases cause the corpse to bloat, and the pressure causes the decayed fluid to purge out of the mouth, nose and anus. The fluids are brown and can look like blood, which often complicates the picture.'

They were all watching and listening grimly. In the mortuary filled with the odours of death, this was not a pleasant topic.

'The gas build-up can become so massive that a body can erupt volcanically when we open it with a scalpel. I've also heard you can light the gas and it burns a beautiful blue, but I've never seen that done.'

I was not trying to be gory or freak them out, but the timing of death was important.

'So you can see that Jason is nowhere even close to advanced putrefaction. This crepitus is still only in his chest, and it's still at quite an early stage.'

'How long do you reckon, Doc?'

That was the burning question.

'I reckon four or five days. Maybe six. No more.'

There was a collective exhalation from the watching men. Then he must have been alive when they were searching and they hadn't found him. No-one likes to fail and these men took their decision to abandon a search-and-rescue damned seriously.

'This is interesting.' I was examining his hands. The detectives gathered around. 'There are no defence or other injuries to his hands, of course, but look how his fingers have dried out. That's mummification.'

The skin was taut, leathery and was darkened to black. They felt hard and there was none of the softening of decay.

'Look at his nails. They look pretty long, but that's because the flesh has shrunk, exposing them. We often see that. It's supposed to be the origin of the myth that your nails keep on growing even after you are dead. And look. The same early mummification is there on his nose, his lips and the right side of his cheek.' I studied the photograph of the scene. 'That would be the side that was exposed to the sun.'

'What does it mean?'

'You only get mummification when the weather is dry. Dry and hot is best, but dry and cool can do it, too. The point is it has to be bone dry.'

I turned to the Dannevirke police officers.

'Can you get me the weather data for the area over the whole period he's been missing?'

They were nodding.

'That would be held by Dannevirke Station. We'll pick that up for you.'

* * *

I could find absolutely no evidence of any injuries or fractures. Jason was well nourished, and even had food in his stomach. Water was evidently not a problem, as he was well hydrated and there was urine in his bladder.

There were two shallow ulcers in his duodenum. They hadn't been there long, maybe a few hours.

'These are stress ulcers,' I decided. 'Curling's, Cushing's or physiological stress ulcers. There're lots of different names. They develop very quickly and they point to a time of significant stress just before death, though they don't tell us what the stress was. Septicaemia, shock or severe injury can all do it. But I don't see any sign of any of those.'

We looked at each other thoughtfully.

'That wraps it up for the time being,' I said. 'There's the toxicology still to come on his blood, urine and stomach contents. That may yet give us the answer. But the important negatives I have established.'

I ticked them off on my fingers.

'One: no injuries. Two: no medical diseases. Three: no evidence of murder. And the timing since death is somewhere between four and six days.'

It was not completely satisfying, but it was something. Jason's body could go back home where he belonged tonight.

* * *

The special investigations began to come in.

I studied the weather data first, looking at the detailed tables and a graph from Dannevirke Station D06212.

'Interesting, 5.8 millimetres of rain on the 13th and 14th of December and then quite a bit more, 43.8 millimetres, on the 17th and 18th. Finally another 12.8 millimetres on Christmas Day. And then no rain right up to when Jason was found nine days later. I think it's too wet until late December for mummification to occur. The temperatures, too, are below 20 or low 20s right up until January 1st, where it climbs to 28 degrees and holds there. The mummification isn't extensive and fits well with the four-to-six-day timeframe, too.'

The toxicology report came from the ESR. Blood, urine and stomach contents were all negative for all drugs, medications and a range of common poisons.

I phoned the ESR scientist and explained our need to get a good fix on the time of death. Could they help?

'In a general way, but it's not scientifically proven. When

we do a gas spectrograph on the blood of decomposed bodies, we get a lot of background signals from complicated alcohols that the bacteria have produced. The longer the period since death, the more decay and the more long-chain alcohols we see.'

'A bit like ageing wine in a cellar,' I guessed. 'The longer you leave it, the more complex esters form which give it textures and flavour.'

'Sort of, although I'm not sure these alcohols would give much flavour!'

'So what did his blood look like?'

'Not too bad. Certainly didn't look as complicated as some I've seen. I can't put a date on it but I'd guess a couple of days, maybe?'

And finally, late in March, the insect report from the entomologist came in the post. It was the first I'd ever seen, and I settled down to read it with interest.

First of all, I found out that I'd stuffed it up. The maggots did indeed need to be killed as soon as collected, just as I had dimly remembered. But not the way I did it. I had put them into neat alcohol. That meant they were preserved, all right, but they had shrunk in the strong liquor and couldn't be accurately measured. Apparently they should have been killed by boiling them in water first, which apparently leaves them *au naturel*. This was embarrassing.

I shuddered. God! Boiling live maggots! That was a bit on the nose.

The maggots apparently were all from the brown blowflies, *Calliphora stygia*, with none from *Calliphora quadrimaculata*, the native blue blowfly. The natives were evidently too slow off the mark to benefit here. I had also picked up a parasite wasp and a rove beetle, both of which were there only as scavengers to feast on the maggots.

I shuddered again. Eating maggots. They can keep that ecological niche!

The weather had been fine for all types of fly throughout the whole of December and January so that didn't narrow things down. I read on.

'It is my opinion that a period of about three to four days has elapsed during which time the body has been present at the scene and available to insects.'

That was about the same time as everything else we'd looked at.

We settled on a time of death somewhere around four to six days prior to when Jason was found. That meant on or around around 30 December. That was long after the official search had been called off, so we could say with confidence that Jason had not been lying exposed on that rocky bed and been missed by the helicopter search crew. More sombrely, though, it meant he had been up there alive and well and the search-and-rescue operation had failed to find him.

It still left us frustratingly nowhere, so far as the cause of death was concerned.

Now we had to face the family at an inquest. The Dannevirke coroner, Stuart Smith, asked me to drive across the ranges, as the extended family was expected to be there. The family were still unhappy with the negative result of the search effort.

I gave my meagre evidence. I didn't know the cause of death. I knew many things that it was not: suicide, murder, injury, catastrophic medical diseases, poisons were all out. But there had clearly been acute stress at the end. The weird ulcers in his duodenum told me so.

Perils in the Bush

But where had Jason been all that time since mid-December? He didn't look as though he had been lost and stumbling around, trying to find his way out. His clothes were tidy and not weather-beaten. He must have been under shelter most of the time. His feet were bare and they were totally uninjured, so he must have been wearing shoes. Where were they? I reckoned they were somewhere close to where we found him.

So what was that final stress caused by? Was it just simple exposure? Heat stroke? Surely not. There was water up there. It wasn't all that hot until the last few days, by which time I thought he was already dead. I had nothing useful to add to the mystery.

With a heavy heart, I gave my opinion that Jason had died of obscure natural causes.

I was dismissed from the witness box and I left to get back across the mountains to my duties. The hearing went on and Stuart had to extend it into a further day so everyone involved could have their say.

* * *

A few years went by and I couldn't get Jason out of my mind. I was satisfied the search-and-rescue operation hadn't missed him lying there, but it nagged at me that we had all overlooked something that might explain his death. One day, I told Jason's story to my retired surgical colleague and friend John Coutts.

'In the Ruahines, you say? In the foothills? That rings a bell.'

Off John went to his attic, stuffed full of surgical notes, papers and memorabilia collected from a lifetime of medicine in the Manawatu.

'Here you are.' John climbed down and thrust a paper at me. 'It happened back in 1961. A bit before your time.'

It sure was. I was only seven at the time.

'It was over Dannevirke way in the Ruahines, pretty much where your chap was found. That's what reminded me. Two young men, 18 and 21 years old, went up there shooting. It was the same time of year too — Boxing Day, in fact, and pretty warm so they were lightly clad. They left coming down until quite late and it was early evening when they did. They couldn't see quite clearly where they were going as it was getting dark and they pushed through quite dense bush. They ran into a bank of tree nettles. Do you know what they are?'

I shook my head. 'I've heard of nettles, but what are tree nettles?'

'*Urtica ferox*,' John said happily. He had an encyclopaedic knowledge of the New Zealand bush. 'It means "Fierce Itch". It's a native found on the fringes of the bush. They grow to two metres and their leaves are covered with rigid stinging hairs, each about six millimetres long. There are patches of them clumped in small localities over several parts of the ranges. Anyway, these blokes were wearing shorts, just like your man Jason. They said they had run into a lot of stinging nettle and it felt like a million needle pricks. Less than an hour later, one of the lads developed a guts ache and couldn't go on. He just lay down and soon became paralysed. He said he had trouble breathing and shortly afterward he became blind, too. His friend managed to get help and they got him out and to the hospital. He died five hours later. His mate developed similar symptoms but not quite as severe and he eventually recovered.'

I was stunned. 'Why the hell haven't we all heard of this?' John shrugged.

'They're known to kill animals, too,' he said, his blue eyes twinkling with amusement. 'Horses are particularly prone and can die quite quickly. They usually have fits and become paralysed. It does something to the nervous system. There was a group of trampers back then who got stung and they had serious incoordination for three days.'

After this conversation, I did some research. Tree nettle may well leave no sign on the skin and its poison, called triffydin is exotic and not well known. It's a great name. It's named after the triffids, moving plants that stung people to death and then ate them, from John Wyndham's famous sci-fi book *The Day of the Triffids*. The ESR wouldn't have found triffydin, because they didn't know to test for it. And death can be very rapid.

Was it a tree nettle that killed Jason? I was quite sure that was the only plausible explanation. Something had killed him and it wasn't murder, suicide, injury, exposure to the elements or any medical disease. In Africa or Australia I would have wondered about a snake bite, but that is one peril we thankfully do not face in New Zealand.

I met with the dignified Chase whanau and their friends to tell them of what I had found and what I thought had happened. I was flabbergasted by what I heard.

Dave is Dannevirke born and bred and is a local farmer, a hunter and a friend of the family who knew Jason well. He had also been a tireless member of the whanau search.

'I knew about the death of the young men by the nettle trees back in 1961,' Dave said. 'I remember my father talking about it. He was involved in their rescue back then. And we hunters know that you have to pull on leggings to protect yourself if you're wearing shorts up there.'

That was a surprise. The nettle danger was therefore known, at least locally, even though the country at large seemed to have forgotten. But it was what came next that made me sit up.

'We found Jason in Nettle Gully. It's a hard way down and ringed by nettles and bloody difficult to get through. I reckoned he was coming back down home and chose the wrong gully. He meant to come down the one a bit further on but made a mistake.'

A mistake. That's exactly what it was.

We believe Jason went into the bush for some time out. I now found out his sleeping bag was missing as was his backpack. His water bottle was found by whanau nearby. He had food, water was plentiful and when he was ready he trekked out. The bush is hard and can be deceptive and he just took the wrong gully.

An accident. Nettle trees were the only plausible cause of death. I was pleased at the outcome. I had never been at peace with Jason for years. His death had never made any sense to me. Now I could put it away, my job done. His story was now told.

But Jason's death does make me wonder that if we didn't know about this particular danger, what other toxic surprises might be out there in the bush that none of us have yet heard about?

Jason Chase. December 2002. Requiescat in pace.

* * *

Perils in the Bush

I did hear about something else pretty toxic out there in the bush, but it wasn't until 15 years later, in mid-November 2017. I was listening to the radio as I shaved that morning.

'Pakistan has unveiled the remains of a 1700-year-old sleeping Buddha in Khyber Pakhtunkhwa province. US Senator Al Franken is accused of groping and forcibly kissing a woman …'

Same old stuff as usual. But then something grabbed my ear.

'Three people have been hospitalised at Waikato Hospital after consuming wild boar meat, believed to have been contaminated by an unknown substance or bacteria. Shibu Kochummen, his wife, Subi Babu, and her mother, Alekutty Daniel, were rushed to hospital after being found unconscious at their Putaruru home on Friday.'

My pathological antennae pricked up.

The emergency services had been phoned by Subi but she collapsed while talking to them. A friend of the family, Joji Vargese, told the radio reporter what he knew of their story. Shibu and some of his friends went hunting for some wild boar. They caught one, cooked it and consumed it. Fortunately, their children had been fed earlier and separately and therefore had a different meal. Apart from the children, the whole family were now unconscious and in a vegetative state.

I listened to this on the way to work. It was extremely odd. What could cause such a thing in New Zealand?

Of course, in seeking an answer to any mysteriously presenting ailment, doctors first turn to the accumulated experience of what we already know. This is our collection of medical evidence painfully garnered since we first became a questioning and scientific society, centuries ago. Most of it is right, but some is rubbish and there is still the odd hole in our knowledge. We have learned much, and with modern genetic probing, we will soon know more.

By the time I reached work, I had decided that paralysis from botulinum — the virulent toxin released by *Clostridium botulinum*, a bacterium that can contaminate food — was the best medical bet. And this is exactly what their doctors did say. That mystery solved, I turned on my microscope that morning, logged into my computer and began to think about my patients of the day who were awaiting their diagnosis. Then Bruce Lockett arrived with a roar.

'Have you heard about the Indian family eating wild pork and getting paralysed? Sounds like "Go Slow", for sure!'

'What's that? I was thinking botulism.'

I love exotic diseases and enthusiastically keep a mental collection of any that come my way. I knew of oddities such as equestrian urticaria on the thighs of ladies who ride horses in the depths of winter, penile pruritus in young men and brachioradial pruritus or itchy arms in middle-aged, fair-skinned golfers and a score of others. But 'Go Slow' was new to me.

'I heard about it at an evening research talk up at Massey a little while back. It's a paralysis affecting hunting dogs up in Northland, mainly. They eat wild boar and there's some unknown toxin in the pig meat that brings it on. It occurs with some, but not all, pigs and no-one knows what they've eaten to cause it. It must be a poison in some seasonal plant because it only occurs now and then and seasonally.'

'What's the pathology? Did your scientist know?' My mind turned inevitably back to Jason's unsolved death and the mysterious tree nettles, of course.

'The poison destroys a cell's mitochondria, apparently.'

Mitochondria are a cell's power plant. With the batteries flat, nothing could work, just like your iPhone when you forget to put it on the charger.

'They end up dying of muscular paralysis.'

'Like polio?'

'Only quicker. And deadlier.'

I looked it up and found that about 20 to 30 dogs are affected every pig-hunting season. It sounded a very plausible cause for the mystery ailment affecting Shibu and his family. Bruce immediately phoned the pathologists at Waikato to tell them about this disease. Others had beaten him to it, and they were now well aware of 'Go Slow'. But there's no lab test and they couldn't be sure. Botulism was still their preferred diagnosis. The treatment is supportive and the same in both cases, anyway: admit the patient to the ICU, put them on a ventilator, keep their fluid and glucose and electrolytes steady, and add in some really powerful antibiotics because it's the bugs that kill, and then wait for time and nature to effect a cure. It's about the same treatment you'd get for a mamba or a cobra bite in Africa — if you made it to a hospital and into an ICU in the first place, of course.

Happily, the family all made it through, albeit with one non-medical and uniquely New Zealand side effect. The Accident Compensation Corporation declined their claim, as they deemed whatever had happened to them not to be an accident.

Whatever.

I do wonder, though, about the unknown perils in our bush. There are 20 known poisonous plants in New Zealand but we really have no idea about what else could be out there. There are tens of thousands of plant toxins throughout the world, both known and unknown. Brush up against one of these somewhere, or even, at a second remove, eat a wild or a farmed animal that once ate one and you too could become a mysterious death. You will become the subject of a coronial autopsy and may well end up unexpectedly in my mortuary.

'Obscure natural causes' is what I shall have to write on your obituary. Because, like you, I won't know what hit you.

And to think you thought you were just out for a day tramp in the mountains!

* * *

'Gerhard Meijer is a hippy.'

'Okay.'

This was interesting. I wasn't sure how many hippies there were left elsewhere in the world, but there weren't a lot around the Manawatu in the late 1980s. I was still very new to New Zealand back then, and I wasn't yet used to uniformed police officers standing in front of me gravely describing the circumstances of a death.

'He's Dutch. Lives at Himatangi Beach. A real loner. Doesn't drink, doesn't hang out with anyone local. Not sure where he gets his supplies from. I asked the local dairy whether they saw anything of him. They reckoned hardly ever. Matches and candles, that was it. No proper tucker at all. It's all a wee bit strange.'

'Why? Maybe he drove into Palmerston or Foxton or somewhere else for groceries?'

The hospital constable shook his head slowly. I suppressed a flash of irritation. I had heaps of work today, and everything about this story seemed to be slow.

Perils in the Bush

'No,' the cop said. 'He has no car, and no friends with a car. So he never took any trips away from Himatangi to buy food. As far as we know. He's been living there a couple of years. So what the hell is he eating? Now he's dead.'

I couldn't see how any of this involved me, but by now my professional interest had been piqued by the sniff of an unusual death.

'How did he die?'

'We don't know. That's the problem. He's dead in the dunes. That's where some locals found him. Dead with not a mark on him. Lying there, but no signs of a struggle or anything. Just dead.'

There was a silence.

'And?'

'He hasn't got a GP. Never seen anyone at all. So no-one will sign a death certificate. The coroner, Mr Hubbard, has asked if you would do an autopsy so we can complete all the necessary paperwork.'

Of course I would do one.

'Shouldn't I at least examine the scene first?'

'No point. He's already here, downstairs in the fridge. Plenty of Himatangi dunes out there and one's the same as the next. No picking which one he came from now.'

'And his house?'

'Not really a house. More of a shack really. Not his. Reckon he just found it empty and moved in. We haven't been able to locate the owner, who has apparently gone to live in Ballarat. No food in his shack at all. A fireplace, a few bits and pieces and a pot with some green crap in it. Looked like slime.'

'Did you bring it?'

'Nah. Chucked it out. No-one wants to see that crap.'

He shrugged his shoulders dismissively.

I really didn't know what to expect from this autopsy.

Gerhard was of indeterminate age though he had a youngish appearance. I thought he was thirty-five or so, but he could have been as much as forty-five. He was ashen blond with no grey hairs that I could see. His skin was a deeply tanned bronze, more what you'd find on a surfer or a lifesaver from an Australian beach than on a man loping around the sandy dunes of the western Manawatu. His skin was unblemished, his teeth were perfect and white and he was finely muscled. There wasn't a gram of fat on him so his muscles were cleanly chiselled out beneath his skin.

'One hundred and sixty-five centimetres!' Bruce Scott called out as he peered at the two-metre-long calliper ruler. The crossbar of the fixed headpiece was hard up against Gerhard's head and Bruce had placed the lower sliding arm hard up against his stiffened feet. The dead obviously can't stand up to measure their height so we measure their length lying down. Likewise, they can't stand on a normal scale, so we wheel them onto a platform scale in the passage leading into our mortuary. The scale has been set so the weight of the gurney is zero and only the patient's weight is recorded. It's their last stop on their way to the table.

'Here you are, weighed in the balance,' Bruce used to intone in a biblical voice as he wrote down the figures in his notebook in the passageway, 'before you are allowed to enter the place where your final outcome will be decided once and for all.'

'What was his weight, Bruce?'

'Only a lightie. Forty-seven point three kilograms. That's about seven and a half stone, Doctor.'

'Thank you, Bruce.'

I'd never quite grasped the system of weights and measures that was widespread in New Zealand back then. Thankfully the stones in which we measured weight have eroded, worn away over the years, leaving the far more intelligible metric kilogram. Although I never hear it any more, Elayne tells me many of her older patients still only know their weight that way.

I looked in the tables. That meant a body mass index of only 18. Pretty underweight, but I had already guessed he wasn't eating much hogget up there in the dunes.

The autopsy was uneventful, really. In fact, it was quite pleasant and easy. All Gerhard's tissues dissected beautifully with each organ hanging cleanly and sweetly, child-like and unlarded with the fatty medallions accumulated in a lifetime of overindulgence. I was amazed. The organs didn't slip from my greasily filmed gloves, escaping my grasp to slop wetly onto the heavy, damp, wooden dissecting board. They were all firm and dry and popped apart like Lego.

And each organ was perfect. His arteries were all soft and perfect, flexible and milky like a lightly steamed squid. I felt along each of his coronary arteries and over his aorta and the huge arteries leading to the brain. There was no trace of fatty atheromatous plaques squeezing out like toothpaste and none of the hard, calcified, diseased reefs built from the savage beatings of arterial disease that I saw so commonly as the fruits of our Western diet.

Pristine. Pliable. Perfect. I was sure they were the best arteries that anyone could find anywhere in the entire world. Yet here he was, dead.

'What's this?' I asked, puzzled.

Bruce came over from where he was pulling the scalp back into position from where I had peeled it forward over the face. He had a suture needle in his fingers and was preparing to stitch it back into position.

He looked at the organ in my hands.

'I think that's the liver, Doctor,' he said.

I looked up at him in irritation. His twinkling eyes gave him away. This dry Kiwi humour took some adjusting to.

'Well done! Correct at first guess.' I thought I would give it back to him. 'But do you know how to "tell" meat?'

'No, Doctor.' Bruce looked at me quizzically.

'Well, I learned in Africa to look at meat and "tell" the species and whether it is diseased or not. It's important for your health, you see. You don't want to eat measled meat, do you? Now does this liver look healthy enough to eat?'

'Never touch it. Liver's crap food, if you ask me, Doctor. But that looks normal to me.'

'Well, it's not okay. I agree with you, I can't see anything wrong but it sure doesn't feel like the liver you get at Woolworths, that's for certain. It's springy. It's got a hard texture to it that feels bad. There's fibrosis here but it's not obvious cirrhosis.'

We saw cirrhosis from alcohol abuse pretty often. This was quite different from that.

But that was all I found. I sent blood for toxicology. The tests were pretty primitive back then: arsenic and alcohol would be about it. No old lace or any other frivolous exotica way back then. And so it proved. There was nothing conclusive to be found, so my accustomed, hopelessly equivocal 'obscure natural causes' report went out to the coroner.

Perils in the Bush

The real answer came only slowly and over some months — decidedly unlike the way scientific answers happen on television shows such as *CSI*, where everything is easy and it's all wrapped up in 40 minutes.

When I first put Gerhard's liver under the microscope, it was like nothing I had seen before.

Fine tendrils of fibrous scarring crept out along the highways and byways of the tissue. The fibrous tendrils looked just like the rootlets of a tree, and just like tree roots lifting and breaking the pavement, the scar tissue filaments had distorted and fractured and plugged the vascular canals of the liver. It looked much like a city after an earthquake, with collapsed buildings and rubble blocking every street. It was obviously very abnormal pathologically, but it wasn't a disease I recognised. I couldn't find a picture in any of the textbooks to match it, either. My colleagues were equally puzzled.

The police eventually brought in more information.

'He's a vegan.' The constable frowned at the word in his notebook.

'What's that mean?' This was 1988, after all. We were still all very naïve.

'He only eats vegetables, Doctor.'

'What vegetables does he eat?'

'None, as we have been able to ascertain. Doesn't grow any or buy any, apparently. But he does collect plants from the dunes and around the bush.'

'What plants? What does he do with them?'

'From what we've been told, it's mainly just weeds and leaves from shrubs. He makes a soup of them. That's all he eats.'

I was disbelieving. I had never heard of anyone living only off wild plants.

'C'mon. That's impossible! He must be having some fries from the local chippie as well, surely?'

He shook his head.

'No way. Not according to the locals. Never gets anything in. Nothing at all.'

Odd diets weren't really mainstream in the '80s as they are today. This was certainly the oddest voluntary diet I had ever heard of. I shook my head in amazement. It didn't seem possible, but it made me think. Was this liver fibrosis due to some strange dietary deficiency?

I cast my mind back, searching for a solution.

I remembered when I was a registrar in training I received a pot of formalin holding about two inches of popliteal artery — the one that pulsates at the back of your knee. This was surgically cut from a 20-year-old woman. I saw that in the middle of the vessel, she had popped up and blown out an aneurysm. It was round and smooth just like a party balloon. I examined it and confirmed what it was, but why was it there at all? Who has ever heard of popping an aneurysm behind your knee?

I could find nothing unusual under the microscope to suggest a cause. But you are what you eat — you have to be, as there's nothing else. The young woman was a ballerina who performed with the Cape Town City Ballet. She was apparently permanently on an unbelievably minimalistic diet designed to keep her weight down. She told us many of them also smoked to suppress their appetites. I suppose they have to be agile and light to be lifted up so elegantly by their dance partners, so their weight is important.

In her case, it was a matter of you become what you don't eat, for she had scurvy. Scurvy, or vitamin C deficiency, was a very common disorder in the age of exploration, when people took slow sailing ships on long expeditions, far from sources of fresh food. But it's practically unheard of in the developed world today. Because she ate so little, the ballerina had serious vitamin C deficiency and this had weakened the walls of her arteries. A dancer threw her skyward and caught her ever so elegantly as she fell, expertly clasping behind her knees. His fingers dug deeply into her popliteal artery and tore its weakened fabric. This started the leak that would in time balloon into her aneurysm. Fortunately, she didn't lose her leg, which was a real possibility, but she certainly would never be a ballerina ever again.

So I had a suspicion that the problem with Gerhard's liver may have had something to do with his unconventional diet, but I was no closer to determining what it might be.

Then, one morning, James came into my laboratory and flicked a medical journal onto my desk. 'Look at this! There's an article in the journal about a vegetarian dying of liver disease after eating comfrey.'

'What's comfrey?' I hadn't heard of this before.

'It's a plant, apparently. Quite common. People take it as a folk remedy. Good for bones, they say. But now it's killed a 26-year-old vegetarian. Toxic to the liver, it seems. It reminded me of your man living up in the dunes.'

I studied the journal closely.

James was right. The pathology in the liver was identical to Gerhard's specimen. His change must have been caused by a toxic plant, and it's a lesson for our times. Such is the backlash against processed and manufactured foodstuffs that an uncritical mythology has arisen about plants generally. If they're natural, they must be good, is the way the reasoning goes. It sounds right but it's so wrong. Many plants produce deadly chemicals. After all, Socrates was executed with hemlock, wasn't he? And that deadly dose he was given in ancient times came from a natural plant, too.

God only knows what Gerhard had grubbed out of the dunes in his short years up there, but somewhere and from some plant that he collected to make his soup, there must have been some with pyrrolizidine alkaloids on board. These chemicals are tasteless and practically undetectable poisons. They are lying in wait in the leaves and fruit of our apparently quiet and gentle bush. My research showed that the seeds of *Crotalaria*, otherwise known as rattlepods, definitely produce these liver toxins. And there may well be plants that are full of other unknown poisons yet to be discovered.

Whatever the precise plant toxins were, they stuffed up Gerhard's liver completely and I reckon they killed him, too. Certainly nothing else did. His arteries were to die for, so to speak, and that is exactly what happened. He simultaneously ate his arteries into perfect health and his liver unto death. And that's what I told the coroner.

It's good advice to stick to the poison-free plants our ancestors ate. After all, that's how they safely came to be our ancestors and how we successfully descended from them in order to be here, today.

Gerhard Meijer. 1988. Requiescat in pace.

My heart aches, and a drowsy numbness pains
My sense as though of Hemlock I had drunk
— John Keats, 'Ode to a Nightingale' (1819)

CHAPTER 13

In My Considered Opinion

When I first came to New Zealand in the 1980s, I found some quaint phrases in autopsy reports that I hadn't come across before. The reports described the positive and negative findings of the autopsy, just as you'd expect. But then there would be a final paragraph which would summarise everything beginning with the phrase 'In my considered opinion'. The last paragraph in a report into a motor vehicle fatality, for example, would say something like: 'In my considered opinion, John Doe died as the result of a fractured skull, a traumatic subarachnoid haemorrhage and underlying cerebral laceration and contusion.' And seemingly as an afterthought, there often used to be the startling phrase added: 'There is no evidence of poisoning leading to this death.'

Who knows how this phrase came to be deemed necessary? Was there a time in our history when poisonings were a dime a dozen? In reality, we only rarely test for poisons. And as most poisons are difficult to detect without specialist toxicology, there were usually no sound scientific grounds for tacking this determination onto the end of a report.

So much for the closing line of the final paragraph.

As I mentioned there was also that wonderful set of words that opened it: 'In my considered opinion …' An opinion is really all that doctors give to their patients, and pathologists are no different. Typically we hear the patient's history, carry out an examination (which is the autopsy for us), send off a few lab tests and put it all together to produce our opinion, which physicians dignify with the name 'diagnosis', which comes from Greek words meaning 'to tell apart'. We pathologists send our reports on to the coroner with our findings so they can determine the cause, the circumstances and the date of death at an inquest. They call this a verdict or a finding but, like our findings, it too is also just an opinion. In each case, another doctor or pathologist may have quite a different opinion, which doesn't mean the first was wrong. It only means you now have two opinions to choose from, and generally you have no way of saying which is right or better than the other.

This is true not only of medicine but also of fields such as the law, economics, social theory and, indeed, just about every field of human endeavour. Some 'pure' sciences such as mathematics may be the exception, but even those may have acquired room for doubt in the age of quantum theories of reality.

In a recent experiment in England, 35 coroners were each sent three cases containing nine complete sets of information, each about a different dead patient. They were asked to reach a verdict on each and justify their finding. Surprisingly, they came up with 12 completely different conclusions, and this range of opinions was found to be solely due to the different personalities of the coroners.

The differences of opinion between coroners seems pretty dramatic in England. For instance, suicide rates vary from a barely credible zero in some regions to an equally mind-boggling 60 per cent of deaths in others, although there is little difference between the regions in most respects. It's just not possible. One of the coroners is getting it wrong, but which one? Perhaps it's both? But that's humanity. Let's be honest, even our best efforts at finding the truth and our fixed beliefs are often just opinions dressed up as fact. Some will be arrived at by random roads and may well be seriously flawed.

Over the years, I have often been asked to give my opinion on a variety of cases and events involving both life and death. They range from the trivial through to others involving murder most foul, but they all tend to be very interesting. They would have to be, I suppose, since someone else has ended up perplexed enough to ask for a second opinion. Some are about living people, some have had an autopsy elsewhere, some never had one and some are just unusual. Some have an answer and some never will.

* * *

'Hi, my name's Sonia. I am phoning you because I read your book, and I can't find anyone else to help me.'

This happens quite a lot. Sometimes the call is from a relative of a patient whose story I have told, sometimes from readers to say they enjoyed the stories, and sometimes from people with interesting stories and problems of their own. Sonia's call proved to be one of the latter.

'What's the problem?'

'Well, it's a bit complicated.'

I sighed. These stories usually are. I settled back, listening.

'I've been found guilty of drink-driving.'

I sighed even more heavily and looked at the overflowing tray of slides waiting for my diagnosis. But I listened on.

'I work at nights as a cleaner. It's a high-end set of holiday apartments in Queenstown. They usually get hired out for a few days or so, not often longer. When they're vacated, I clean them. Well, I had eight or nine to clean and I started at 7 p.m. The bathrooms all have enclosed showers and we clean those using alcohol steam units. Do you know them?'

'No, never heard of them. What are they?'

'They spray out hot methylated spirits and water in a mist. They're fantastic for cleaning showers. I always use them. It took me two and a half hours to steam all the showers. I know that because I photographed all of them on my phone and sent them to my supervisor at 10.30 p.m. to show that the work was properly done. I always do that. They were spotless.'

I wondered where this was going.

'It was evening, so I had a glass of white wine while I was working, but that's all. I locked up and left just after 10.30 p.m. At the first roundabout, the police stopped me and breathalysed me. It was positive. I couldn't believe it. I had a blood test, too.'

'What was the level?'

'High. It was 192 milligrams.'

'Mmm, that's very high. You're sure you only had one glass?'

'I promise you it was just one. That's why I can't believe it. I wasn't drunk. It's not possible. I think I got it from the spray. Can you get it that way?'

I'm not sure why, but I believed her story. Her tone, the way she told the story, had a ring of truth. I was interested. I thought I would investigate it further.

Sonia told me she is a slight young woman and not really used to drinking.

'I told my lawyer what happened, but he said it was better just to plead guilty. So I did. I lost my licence for a year but I've come to terms with that. It's just that I think it's all so unfair. I asked them if it was possible that it was inhaled alcohol, but they said no, it was impossible. They told me there was no further testing possible.'

This was interesting. I decided to check this story out.

'Where's your blood sample? At the ESR lab, I would guess?'

The equipment checked out. It did use hot methylated spirits in a vapour spray. Apparently the hot meths had the double advantage of removing the fat-laden skin cells that smear on shower walls as well as flushing away the limestone salts deposited by hard water. In the course of my research, I learned that methylated spirits is not methanol as it was in days gone by. Now it's ethanol — same as the active ingredient in your evening glass of wine — although it's still coloured a toxic purple and it's still fatal to drink it at those concentrations.

But can you get drunk by inhaling alcohol? Well, it's amazing but true that there are bars that specialise in breathable booze. These tout it as the ultimate experience. There's one on the south bank of the Thames where you get to inhale gin and tonic vapour from a humidifier. You suck it into your lungs, where it's absorbed and passes directly to the brain, supposedly avoiding the detoxifying liver. You're allowed in the room for a maximum of one hour: any longer and you will get too drunk!

'My God!' I exclaimed to the pathologists in the lab. 'You can get drunk without a drop touching your lips!'

'But that wouldn't change the law, would it?' they argued. 'You'd still be over the legal limit for driving and drunk in charge?'

'That's true,' I had to admit. 'But surely it's a mitigating factor to put before the judge. Just imagine! Drunk as charged, but only because of an unforeseen work hazard. What jury could resist that?'

But Sonia's case was dead and gone, it seemed. The charge had been laid, admitted to and the penalty imposed. She had sucked it up and got on with her life. But I couldn't help but wonder. If her story were true, was it a fair punishment?

We know all about drinking alcohol and exactly how it pushes up your blood-alcohol levels. Human beings have been knocking it back for thousands of years, and its effects are pretty well known. In the last few decades, measuring the levels of alcohol in the bloodstream of drivers has become a matter of some precision. Yet, apparently, there are surprises still to be had.

On 2 January 2017, Janice Tua breastfed her two-month-old daughter Sapphire, one of two premature twins. Sapphire was found dead in her cot soon afterwards. Sapphire's autopsy showed nothing physically amiss. According to the coroner, Debra Bell, as advised pathologically the formal cause of death was unascertained. Sapphire had blood level of over 300 milligrams per 100 millilitres, which is six times the adult driving limit! It turned out that Janice had drunk 18 cans of pre-mixed bourbon and Coke during the New Year's Day holiday, and in the absence of any other source it is believed that Sapphire had become intoxicated downstream through the breast milk. Comments were made at the inquiry about the inadvisability of drinking alcohol in breast feeding mothers. We always suspected that alcohol could get into milk, but I for one would never have believed it could do so to this sort of level. I was not alone in thinking so. Dr Jack Newman, in his handout 'More Breastfeeding Myths', says: 'As is the case with most drugs, very little alcohol comes out in the milk. Prohibiting alcohol is another way we make life unnecessarily restrictive for nursing mothers.' And breastfeeding advocate organisation the La Leche League International agrees.

So what is happening here? Comments in the inquiry suggest one thing; the scientists in the field say completely another. Both are, of course, opinions and not proven facts.

Could it be that there is more than we know about how alcohol affects breast milk? Could it perhaps become preferentially concentrated in some mothers' milk, but not others? We should scientifically find out for certain, if only to make sure that we all know the truth and justice is well served.

We certainly are in the blind about vaping alcohol. All of the medical papers concerning alcohol inhalation are about alcohol-containing hand gels, and they have been found to have minimal effects on blood alcohol. Sonia's exposure seems to be at a different level altogether, and I'm not sure we have heard the end of this particular problem yet. Niall Campbell, an English specialist in alcohol addiction, is right in expressing his horror at recreational alcohol vaping. 'The last thing this country needs is another way of ingesting alcohol!'

* * *

The opinions I have been asked vary in their importance as well as in the level of interest they hold. Some have been trivial, others significant, and some just plain delightful, teaching me something I never knew before.

One day a senior forensic pathologist handed me a slide.

'Is this anisakiasis?'

'Anisakiasis?'

My brain was a huge black hole. What the hell was that? I had only the vaguest recollection of the name. It wasn't anything I had ever come across in Africa or New Zealand. Wasn't it something to do with fish?

I looked at the slide under my microscope. There was a slice of small bowel and sitting in the muscle coat was a grotesque parasite that was certainly a larva of some sort. A quick reference to the *Atlas of Tropical Diseases* revealed an identical photograph. It was an *anisakis* larva, beyond any doubt.

'Where in hell has this come from?'

My mind switched back to my early days in Africa where I had made an intensive study of parasites. Although anisakiasis was not found off the African coast, I remember reading it occurred in the North Sea. To be looking at this sample under my microscope in Palmerston North, it surely had to be from an immigrant.

'Is this someone from Holland? Or somewhere in northern Europe?'

But no. The victim was a Kiwi who had presented with abdominal pain initially diagnosed as appendicitis. That was pretty typical, I learned. So was his subsequent death.

This affliction arises from an infestation of round worms that happily live in the stomach of dolphins and whales and sea lions. The parasite survives and spreads by passing from one sea mammal to another in the flesh of the raw fish they dine on. I have seen a dolphin's stomach lining crawling with the adult worms in the Parasitological Museum in Tokyo. Don't worry if you've never heard of the Parasitological Museum. It's a pretty niche interest.

Anisakis is a 'spill-over' parasite. It doesn't usually affect people, because we just don't swim around the open ocean eating raw fish. But suppose you *do* go and eat raw fish. Well, now. That changes everything.

If ingested alive, it does all sorts of horrible things to people, and it can also kill you, and suddenly. The larvae first burrow into your bowel, where they hunker down in the muscle of the gut. The inflammation they cause is often misdiagnosed as appendicitis. But then they may suddenly release some of their crap into your circulatory system and that causes sudden shock, anaphylaxis (a severe allergic reaction) and often death. Sometimes you live and sometimes you don't. The patient whose slide I was viewing clearly didn't.

I love sushi. You probably do, too. Predictably, anasakiasis used to be common in Japan, the home of sashimi. The Dutch have always eaten raw fish, too. I was appalled as a young man the first time I ever saw rollmops, which is their raw, pickled, wrapped-over herrings. I thought they looked disgusting, just like a roll of python skin, and who knows: there may have been an ancient, atavistic instinct telling me to keep away, because sometimes rollmops hold death in their fishy flesh. Dutch herrings occasionally carry the spawn of the *anisakis* worm buried in their muscles. For years, this was a big problem for the Dutch, but they found a way to polish these worms off. All fish that were to be eaten raw must be frozen at -20 degrees centigrade for at least 24 hours.

This sorts the little buggers out by freezing them to death. The Japanese eliminated the disease the same way.

But where the hell had this one come from, and what was it doing here in New Zealand? I looked up the story of this disease. As it's well known in Japan, it clearly does live in the Pacific as well as in the North Sea. So it's not surprising to find that the parasites live, happily breeding their families, here in our inshore fish and marine mammals.

This means we're at risk too. This was news to me, and caused me to rethink what I had come to believe was okay to eat. Some of our pathologists now refuse to eat raw fish in our restaurants. That's probably rational, but I still order it regularly. I do love sushi, and I sometimes wonder if I wouldn't have been better off enjoying it in complete ignorance.

* * *

I have only once been asked for an opinion from overseas, and the occasion has stuck in my mind. The inquiry came from London, where an inquest was to be heard in the Coroner's Court.

The police wanted a young Jamaican man — let's call him Jerome — to help them with their inquiries into a number of minor crimes that had been committed in their local area. The constables on the beat were briefed to keep their eyes open for him. It wasn't so serious a matter that there was a warrant out for his arrest: all they were supposed to do was ask him politely to come down to the station and answer a few questions.

A pair of constables spotted him and approached him. He saw them and ran. Only he knows why. Maybe he did know the answers to the questions the police wanted to ask him, but who can tell?

But as the tiniest pebble rattles down moving another and another and eventually creates a landslide, things now gained their own momentum. Jerome ran as fast as he could, and the police chased him. Of course they did. Dogs are much the same with cats and cars: it's instinctive, really. They caught him after about half a kilometre, no more. Not really that far for a young man to run.

One of the constables grabbed him from behind and pulled him to a stop, holding him tightly by his clothing. To his shock, Jerome went limp, like a dead weight. It didn't take the policeman long to realise that this is exactly what he had suddenly become.

Jerome had died, and technically he was in custody: only just in custody and only just dead, but still dead in custody nonetheless. This could prove a big problem.

The evidence was contradictory. The constable was certain he had grabbed Jerome by his shirt alone and hauled him up short. That was all that had happened. Other witnesses were equally sure a heavy headlock was applied for a protracted period. That happens quite often, too, I suspect.

Who could say who was telling the truth? Emotions were running high, as you might expect.

An autopsy was ordered. The coroner was going to investigate.

It turned out Jerome had an enlarged heart — 625 grams, which was really quite big for a young man weighing 74 kilograms (or almost 12 stone, as the English pathologist put it). I would have expected the maximum weight of the heart of a man the size and physical condition of Jerome to be no more than 300 grams. That meant his heart was swollen to more than twice its normal size.

Why was that? Jerome had an interesting medical background. He was British-born, but his parents were of Jamaican origin. That meant his ancestors had carried the ancient genetic seeds of his distant African heritage across the middle passage hundreds of years ago to the West Indies, and then latterly his mother and father brought them to the English shores. Some of those genes were useful in Africa, where malaria is endemic. Those carrying these genes survived where others did not. For Jerome had abnormal red blood cells, which literally curled up and died when malaria parasites tried to feast on them, a condition known as sickle cell disease. This tended to stop the fatal infection in its tracks — a useful attribute in Africa, but redundant in Europe.

Unfortunately the red cells' response in SCD carriers is not specific to the malarial parasite. They will carry out exactly the same self-destructive implosion for a huge number of ridiculous reasons that wouldn't affect you or me. The technical term is 'haemolysis', and it's where the sufferer's red cells smash more or less like a large pile of plates dropped on a stone kitchen floor. We've all heard that happen now and then in restaurants: it makes just as much of a mess in the body as it does in the kitchen. I was asked for an independent opinion of the significance of this feature of Jerome's genetic heritage and gave it by phone.

'Well,' I said, 'I think he has had long-term, severe sickle cell haemolysis, so his heart is enlarged, probably from anaemia resulting from the break-up of his blood. Because his blood had an impaired capacity to carry oxygen, his heart needed to work twice as hard to make up for it. That's already a very serious state of affairs in a young man. But then, on top of this, he has run fast and hard, closely pursued by the police. Nobody disagrees that he clearly didn't want to be caught or to talk to them. So he was fearful. And excited, of course. And that means lots of adrenaline pumped out.'

Adrenaline is the hormone that gears you up for fear, flight or fight, and it can have a rare and unexplained effect. I had seen slides of Jerome's heart, and the answer — or at least part of the answer — was plain to see. I had examined the slides with my registrars.

'It's cardiac muscle and there is obvious nuclear enlargement, confirming the heavy heart weighed at autopsy. But look at that! What do you see?'

The heart muscle fibres were crunched up as if in a cramp, tight frazzled bands marching in regular columns along each cell.

'It's contraction band necrosis!' the registrars sang out. They saw it and recognised it at once. They were correct. I was proud of them.

This is an unusual finding at autopsy. I first saw it in Africa 40 years ago when a veterinary pathologist showed me the heart of a gemsbok that was being chased by hunting dogs and had apparently dropped dead during the chase without injury.

'It's contraction band necrosis,' he told me. 'We see it quite often in kills in the wild. We think it's from excess adrenaline pumped out in the prey from the fear of the chase. There's just so much adrenaline that the heart muscle just goes into overdrive and it fuses solid.' I know contraction band necrosis has now been studied much more closely. I am not sure this is the whole story, but that's what I first heard 40 years ago and I reckon it still seems right.

The Quick and the Dead

'So,' I continued in giving my opinion over the phone, 'I think Jerome had a badly damaged heart brought on from his sickle cell disease and then when he ran away, he experienced a massive adrenaline overdrive, which caused a heart attack of the "contraction band" type.'

'Could this type of heart attack occur with a police neck lock, such as some witnesses allege they saw?'

'Yes, I suppose it could, although when a neck lock leads to death it is more usually because of neck compression. My opinion is neutral as to the events that occurred during or immediately before the contraction band heart attack happened. That cannot be deduced from this slide. But the heart is certainly the immediate cause of death.'

That is so often our position as pathologists, for we must be honest. What it did mean was that in the light of Jerome's enlarged heart problem, the constables' story of his sudden and unexpected death is quite plausible. Jerome might well have died suddenly with minimal restraint.

What do you think?

* * *

Frankly, we were sick of murders in the Manawatu.

They just kept coming our way at a rate way out of proportion to a population our size. Maybe the stars or something get out of alignment and there's an aberration: whatever it was, we just wanted it to end. But it wasn't to be.

I woke up early on the morning of Tuesday, 4 January 2005, only to find it had happened again. The holiday was over and today was back to work for me. My family were all still asleep as I listened to the seven o'clock news.

'An elderly woman living in Marton in the Rangitikei was found apparently murdered in a burglary gone wrong. Police have cordoned off the scene and are investigating.'

The details were sparse. We weren't on duty for homicides in Palmerston North that day. An American forensic pathologist, George E. Thomas, who was doing a locum in Wellington, travelled up to investigate, and nor did I envy him. It was a horrible story.

Mona Morriss was a delightful 83-year-old, much loved by her nine children, 28 grandchildren and 19 great-grandchildren. They were the fruits of a rich life, one well lived. Mona resided alone, caring for herself in comfortable independence.

Everyone was outraged at this brutal and callous attack. It was the murder of a defenceless, lovely lady, but worse was to come, for the police speculated that there were features that pointed to a sexual attack.

I wasn't involved, but I sensed there was something odd in the wording of the police statement. Why didn't they know for sure? They had investigated the scene, after all, and there had been an autopsy. Surely there either was a sexual attack or there wasn't?

Things were even less clear after Detective Sergeant Tim Smith, who was part of the investigation team, spoke out.

'There is a sexual aspect to the crime scene that police need to consider,' he said. 'It's likely only when the killer is caught that we will know the personal motivations and action described.'

How mysterious. What was the problem? I wondered.

Six months went by with no progress, although during that time the story changed and it was confirmed there had been no sexual attack during the murder. It was a time of immense frustration for the family. Other murders intervened. A couple were knifed to death in Feilding, but resolution was rapid, as the murderer was caught on independent CCTV, no doubt to his chagrin and perhaps to everyone else's complete surprise. But for Mona, there was nothing to show for a long, long investigation.

At last, the news broke that the police had made a breakthrough and arrested 'a person of interest'. I heard only snippets in passing about this, as the murder was being investigated pathologically in Wellington and by a Whanganui-based CIB team. Although I was interested to hear the case was moving along at last, the details largely passed me by.

Then I got a call from Tim Smith.

'Could you review the Mona Morriss case and give your opinion to the court?'

It was more than two years later. This request came as a complete surprise.

'The original forensic pathologist, George Thomas, was only here doing a locum and has since returned to the United States. He can't make it for the trial but we'll need a pathologist to present the evidence and answer the cross-examination. Can you do it?'

I thought hard.

'I'll need to see everything. All the scene photographs and George's autopsy report and his notes, too, if I have to lead the evidence.'

Tim collected it all and I was given a huge file of photographs and notes of the scene, of Mona's body and her autopsy, the interior environs of her home on Wellington Road, the luminol testing of the rooms for blood and of all the rifled cupboards and drawers.

I studied it all and gradually put together the likely sequence of events.

'First, there was the physical attack. Mona was standing facing her assailant,' I later explained to Tim in person. 'The first blow to the left side of her head knocked her spectacles flying to where they were found a good distance from her body. There were then three more hard, but not massive, blows. One was below the right ear, dislodging an earring. One was to the face, fracturing the bone around the orbit of the eye. Then there was a bigger hit to the left side again — sort of a one-two, one-two, probably with the fists.'

'So not a boot, then? Not a kick?'

'I don't think so. The tissue injury is not as great as a kick, though I agree there is a fracture to the underlying skull. But I think there was also a kick. Look at this.'

I pointed to a photograph of Mona's right shin.

'This is geographically distant from the head injuries and is isolated. It's a superficial abrasion. I think it was a kick put in at the same time as the punches.'

The picture I had in my mind was of a fast and frenzied attack, fists and feet flailing.

'I had wondered if the shin abrasion might be from Mona falling to the ground but there's nothing near her body that could have done this. Of course, she would have been unconscious from the very first blows and fallen to the ground, lying on her back. There the killer moved in, opened her blouse and plunged a knife six times into her chest over her heart. It was a murder carried out with intent and great vigour. Each of the wounds alone were individually fatal and with six there was no possibility of survival.'

'Anything else to add?'

'There are no defence wounds to be seen. Mona did not fight back. I guess that fits with the scenario that I am describing of her being unconscious.'

I paused.

'There is one odd thing,' I added. 'I see the killer has carefully covered Mona's body with the bedclothes. Is that right?'

There was affirmative nodding.

'That's very odd. I've never seen that before. Usually murderers are callous, uncaring bastards and just leave their victims where they fall, or sometimes, even worse, mutilate them. This seems to show some sort of oddly misplaced compassion, especially after such a brutal killing. It's almost as if they were sorry for what they'd done. Maybe it was shame. They couldn't bear looking at the results of their attack.'

'Did you know we have arrested and charged a woman with the murder?'

I looked at him in surprise.

'No, I hadn't caught up with that. What's her background? Does she know the victim?'

Tim shook his head.

'No, not at all. No connection. She's a 43-year-old career burglar with 86 previous convictions. Her name is Tracy Goodman and we've got her locked up serving seven years for burglary at the moment, so she's not going anywhere fast. She targets the elderly living alone, often when they're out. Sadly, Mona was at home and I guess she surprised Goodman in the act of breaking in.'

'Why did she have to kill her? Does she usually resort to violence? I suppose she'd been seen and could be identified?'

'No, the resort to violence is new. She's never done anything remotely like this. She's a bad'un, okay — into drugs and theft — but no, murder's not her way, so far. And yes, we also think she did it to avoid being identified.'

There was nothing further to be said. It was a matter of waiting for the trial later in the year.

But then another aspect arose. It was two months later and Tim called again. 'Can you give us some information on the type of knife used? We haven't found the weapon, but a number of knives have been handed in during the inquiry.'

I had been wondering when this particular question was going to come up. It's always a difficult one to handle, as so many of the questions that get asked of pathologists are. Modern forensic lore tells us to keep to a description of the wounds alone and let them speak for themselves. We are urged not to speculate as to intent if we value our reputations. We are told never to speculate on the sequence in which the injuries were inflicted. Some textbooks say that the actual wounds are best used to confirm or deny eyewitness accounts. That may well be the safest course, but I happen to believe that's not particularly useful to a jury. And a fat lot of good that would be in this case. There were no eyewitnesses: only Mona herself was still there to tell us her story.

I could find only one rational explanation for what I could see from the scene and from Mona's injuries, so that is the scenario I had described. But to identify the knife used from the wounds alone is tricky. The problem is that the appearance of any stab wound depends not only on the type of knife, but also upon the many, various and vigorous movements of both attacker and victim in a knife fight. In short, any knife could, if used in a certain way, produce virtually any pattern.

This makes it fertile ground for defence lawyers to discredit any interpretation you might give.

'I'll see what I can do but I can't promise that I'll be able to say anything useful.'

The evidence, however, did seem to point to a common-sense conclusion.

There were six wounds to examine. They showed the blade was between 18 and 30 millimetres wide. Three showed an identical pattern, with a three-millimetre blunt edge and a sharp, incised opposite edge. That is pretty much the cross-sectional appearance and dimension of any common kitchen carving knife.

George Thomas had measured the depth of the stabbings and these showed the knife was at least 8 centimetres and up to 11 centimetres long. Of course, that is only a minimum measurement, as the blade may not be (and usually isn't) plunged in right to the hilt.

My opinion was in favour of a carving knife. It could have been something different, but I thought it was unlikely to be anything much different. Anything else I could think of would be hard to fit into the wounds we had found.

'This has become important, Doctor,' I was told. 'Can you come to the court for a conference?'

This was different from the usual course of events.

'Why? I mean, of course I can. But why? Surely the facts aren't contentious?'

'Someone else has been identified as a possible murderer.'

I was lost for words.

'Was it a freely given confession?'

It was. That was always supposed to be the best possible evidence.

'Has it changed anything? I mean, does the information from the confession fit the events and the scene?'

'We've been given a knife.'

I drove over to Whanganui the next morning and presented myself at the High Court. The trial of Tracy Goodman for murder was under way. We met in a conference room. Tim Smith was there, of course, as well as the Crown prosecutor, Andrew Cameron, and the defence lawyer, Mike Antunovic. According to the rules of discovery, the potentially dramatic development in the case — the confession and the production of the alleged murder weapon — had all been disclosed to the defence team, in the interests of fairness.

I explained my findings as to what I believed the knife to be and why I thought so. I pointed out the features on the photos of Mona's wounds. Tim pulled out a brown envelope, dug his hand in and brought out a knife then handed it to me.

'Could that be the knife?'

It was a rather battered letter opener made of a coloured metal similar to brass. The blade was a stiletto shape, quite blunt, about 10 to 12 millimetres wide and maybe 10 centimetres long.

I studied it carefully and then looked up. Legal and police faces looked expectantly back at me. I shook my head. 'I cannot conceive of any way that this knife could possibly have caused the injuries that Mona Morriss sustained.'

I sensed the tension draining from the room. The lawyers leaned back, nodding at each other. I think we were all relieved to avoid a pointless distraction in what all agreed was a serious trial.

Subsequently, a 15-year-old was charged with making a false complaint. The police had wasted two days investigating his claims that he knew who the killer was. He had an elaborate story which took a lot of unravelling. It all proved to be imaginary and the toerag was referred to Youth Aid.

I didn't even have to give my second-hand evidence, because George Thomas found he could get back from the States, after all, and he presented his findings in person. George phoned me later.

'Thank you so much for your work on the case. I read your evidence and I agree with all the opinions you have given. It's exactly what I said in court.'

Tracy Goodman was found guilty and sentenced to 19 years without parole. This is the longest sentence ever given to a woman in New Zealand. The general opinion around here was that she deserved it, for sure. No-one, let alone an older person, should be the victim of so callous an act. Despite the compassionate use of blankets Goodman used to cover Mona's violated body, I am inclined to agree.

George had an interesting view on that aspect of the case, too.

'I am aware of this phenomenon of covering the body with sheets or bedding happening in the States. It's mainly done by women killers, though it does occur with family murders and in murders committed by gay men also.'

Mona Morriss. 3 January 2005. Requiescat in pace.

CHAPTER 14

Fit to Burst

Hemi Gilberg had a multitude of problems for an 18-year-old.

He was a voracious eater and was thought to be 150 kilograms, which was well up there and easily met the definition of morbid obesity. One consequence of this was that he had developed type 2 diabetes. He also suffered from schizophrenia and was receiving monthly injections to control the symptoms. He had made one half-hearted attempt at suicide a couple of years previously, but now that he was on medication, that seemed to be behind him. He had a history of minor criminal episodes but this seemed to be behind him, too. He lived alone and didn't really have any outside interests other than gaming on PlayStation.

The policeman who was giving me the patient's history paused. I didn't know him: he was from Whanganui, and was plainly a details man. Normally, the history was quite light on specifics.

As if his future wasn't challenging enough, Hemi was also a heavy user of synthetic cannabis. He had been into rehabilitation half a dozen times, too, but so far had not been able to break the habit.

'I see. I suppose he's dead and you want an autopsy?'

It was 9.15 on a Wednesday morning and I tried to cut to the chase. But the policeman was not to be hurried.

'Earlier the district nurse called to give him his monthly injection,' he continued at the same measured pace. 'He wasn't compliant on his pills so he was put on paliperidone. That's an anti-psychotic. It's spelled p-a-'

'Yes, yes,' I interrupted. 'I know what it is. Carry on, please.' At this rate I'd be here until lunchtime.

'Well, the nurse took his blood pressure and it was high. She thought he looked pretty crook so she said she would stop by later in the day to check up on him. She was very shocked to find him dead and is blaming herself for not doing something earlier. His brother called by about mid-morning and found him lying on the floor. He had vomited everywhere and it had gone halfway across the room and splashed high up on the wall.'

'Projectile vomiting,' I mused, really to myself.

'What's that, Doctor?'

I sighed. I really should learn to just shut up and listen. 'It's forceful vomiting that gets hurled a long way. It usually means an obstruction between the stomach and duodenum. You see it quite often in infants but sometimes in adults, too. At Hemi's age, it's more likely to be due to a toxin or an infection.'

'Thank you, Doctor. I've written that down. There was a bag of synthetic cannabis lying next to him as well as a pipe containing the drug. It had been lit and presumably smoked. There was no suicide note to be found.'

I thought I had more than enough of the story to be getting on with, but I was only able to get away by promising to contact the constable immediately if I needed any further information.

Hemi was downstairs waiting for me in the mortuary. I changed into scrubs and my surgical gown, pulled on gloves and boots and went into the dissection room. I stopped and stared. I just couldn't help it.

Hemi was big, very big. He still lay on the trolley, as he was too large to transfer to the gurney.

'My goodness! What's his weight?'

'He's 175 kilograms. Height 175 centimetres,' Pat answered. 'Exactly a kilogram for each centimetre. We'll have to do the autopsy on the trolley since we can't really get him over to the table.'

One hundred and seventy-five kilograms. That was a body mass index of 57. Definitely morbidly obese. I walked around him. His abdomen was round and protuberant and his chest was like a huge wine barrel, too.

'It's hard to tell, but isn't his bowel distended? I mean disproportionately to the rest of him.' I percussed the skin which was drawn tight as a drum. It sounded tympanic, almost hollow. 'Sounds like he's full of air or gas.'

Pat was watching me. He nodded in agreement. 'His gut does look bigger than the rest of him.'

We got to work. Pat took up his scalpel and cut the usual Y-front incision into the skin of the chest with the stem of the Y extending down the midline of the abdomen to reach his crotch. He sliced deeply and confidently as he had so many times before. In most patients, there is a layer of fat beneath the skin and Pat slices straight through that onto the hard bone of the sternum and ribs beneath. Not this time. The incision peeled open showing centimetres of yellow fat right down to the limit of the cut. There was no sign of the chest wall. Pat looked up at me.

'Better go deeper.'

And he did. But still there was just more and more fat and the cut was already 20 centimetres deep.

'He's hiding in there somewhere, Pat. Keep cutting in.'

At 33 centimetres deep the fat layer ended and we finally found the body inside. Way down there was the breastbone. And here was the midline tendon binding the muscles of the abdominal wall to each other. Pat slit the tendon to open the cavity and all hell burst forth.

Wet hawsers of massively dilated bowels exploded under pressure out of the body cavity and spilled like coils of a pinkish-grey python down either side of the trolley, almost to the floor. They were bloated with gas and fluid.

'My God, it's massive bowel obstruction! Both small and large bowels! What on earth has caused that?'

I knew I had to work my way from one end to the other of all 23 feet of small bowel and then five feet of colon and rectum to find the cause of the obstruction. Could it be a hidden cancer causing the blockage? A volvulus, or twist of the colon, was more probable at Hemi's age, though. I had a feeling that I would find nothing there, because I thought this was going to be a paralytic ileus. That's what happens when the gut just stops moving and blows up with gas and fluid. It's usually because a toxin or an infection poisons and paralyses the gut's nerve supply.

It was frustrating work. The bowels were slippery and kept slithering away, and as I moved from side to side of the trolley to follow them, I kept dropping them and losing my place. Then I would have to start again. I could see that Pat was amused but I was becoming increasingly irritable.

The task reminded me of a story told by Bob McCully, who was an American veterinary pathologist I had worked with in Africa. He had to do autopsies on a couple of elephants and with the first he had made the mistake of opening the abdomen first. The guts had poured out until they were piled more than shoulder high. He kept slipping and sliding through the piled-up guts until he was drenched in rank-smelling fatty fluid and under incessant attack by swarms of flies.

'Leave the gut until last.' I will always remember Bob's hard-learned lesson, which he passed on in the unlikely event that I was ever asked to autopsy an elephant. Today, I was having a rather similar experience.

I discovered Hemi's stomach was also hugely distended by gas and two litres of creamy chyme. He had been eating up big before death. Only his duodenum was of normal size. All of his small and large guts were bloated by vast amounts of gas and fluids. As I had expected, there was no cancer or adhesion or hidden, entrapped hernia blocking the gut.

This was functional. Something toxic had paralysed his entire gut. A paralytic ileus.

This may not have been a mechanical blockage, but it was easily enough to kill him just through fluid loss and the resulting dangerous changes to his sodium and potassium electrolytes. But there was more to this death than paralytic ileus alone.

The relentless pressure of swollen loops of bowel tightly trapped within the abdomen had rigidly splinted his diaphragm high up into his chest. Hemi needed his diaphragm to move freely just to be able to breathe. I could see that all that would have been pumping the air in and out of his lungs were the smaller rib muscles of the chest, expanding and contracting his ribcage.

Those rib muscles, too, were in big trouble.

The weight of the fat coating the chest wall compresses and splints them, too, so the ribs can't move freely up and down. This inability to breathe in and out deeply causes another common problem in the morbidly obese. They can't breathe, so their blood oxygen levels drop. This causes the arteries to the lung to become hypertensive and the right side of the heart becomes strained and thickened and begins to fail.

Hemi's blown-up gut together with his obesity simply suffocated him to death. That was the cause of death.

Pat crunched the rib secateurs through the ribs and collarbones on either side of the sternum and pulled it out with an effort. It was really difficult working in the dark depths of a fat-lined cavity. The heart and lungs followed.

I looked down into the empty chest cavity. It looked tiny, but that was just an optical illusion: the cavity was the normal size, of course, but it just seemed small and out of proportion compared with the enormous pannus of fat wrapped around it.

'It almost looks like there is a small person inside trying to get out.'

But what caused the bowel to become paralysed? It was that dilatation in the first place that precipitated the cascade that had led to his death.

'I'm betting it'll be the synthetic cannabis that's caused this. I need his blood and urine to go to the ESR lab for testing.'

Pat nodded. 'I've already taken it.' Of course he had. He was always one step ahead.

Synthetic cannabis: the current scourge of the streets and a potent cause of sudden death. Hemi was my first case, although he wouldn't be my last. For a time, the sale of synthetic cannabis was legal. But as the harm it was doing became obvious, it was banned. Trouble is, of course, you can't just stick the genie back in the bottle and re-cork it. The production and sale simply went underground. Back when I met Hemi, it was still very new, so I set out to find out all I could about these drugs. It's pretty sobering.

They are designer drugs and there are thousands of them and the active compounds are all different so they can be impossible to test for. It seems they can be 85 times more potent than THC, the psychoactive chemical in marijuana. The effects are variable, probably because they're just run up any old way in gang houses or who knows where. There is no control of production. Basically the chemicals are dissolved in a solvent and sprayed any old how onto dried plant material which is then smoked. No-one knows or cares what concentration should or shouldn't be used and so it's not surprising that there is a huge range of strengths. Some samples are ten times stronger than others!

The popular one in New Zealand is called AMB-FUBINACA and it arrived early in January 2016. It hasn't proved to be a Happy New Year present for New Zealand. Over 45 New Zealanders have died since mid-2017 from these drugs, and more are dying all the time. People have fits on these drugs, some get kidney failure and many are just found dead. In New York City in the summer of 2016 FUBINACA, sold as K2, caused a real-life zombie apocalypse. Thirty-three people were afflicted like zombies with blank stares and slow responses, were unable to stand and many became unconscious. They were even shown on TV One news staggering mindlessly around the streets.

Then it happened in Auckland, too. In July 2017, there was a spate of 15 deaths from FUBINACA. I heard that crystals of the drug could be seen coating the carrier plants so it must have been a really strong batch — strong enough to be serially fatal to a host of people.

When will people learn? Why would anyone in their right mind take any chemical which is of completely unknown type or strength and which is known to have deadly side effects? They do, and of course, that's how I come to meet these lost souls in my professional capacity.

I searched everywhere, but I could find absolutely no mention of paralytic ileus caused by synthetic cannabis. So reluctantly I conceded I must be wrong in my early assumption that the guilty party was synthetic cannabis. What did kill Hemi, then?

I turned to investigate his monthly anti-psychotic injection of clozapine.

And there, finally, was the surprising answer. It was hidden away in the small print that reels off the complications — the side effects — of every medicine, but it was there nonetheless.

'The drug can paralyse the nerves of the gut and cause a gastric and gut dilatation,' I read. 'In extreme cases, there may be a significant paralytic ileus and bowel obstruction.'

It is very rare and there was only one case reported in the medical journals, although another 30 have been recorded with the relevant adverse drug reaction registers but never published in journals.

Poor Hemi. He had so many social and medical issues to deal with and to die of a rare side effect of his prescribed medication is heartbreaking in so young a man. We do much right in medicine and in our society, but there are still so many things that we end up handling quite poorly. He was a case in point. Hemi needed and deserved a break, although I know it's hard to see how that might have happened.

We see the tragic results of both social and medical failures at every level daily in the mortuary. Would that we could all learn from these mistakes and make them and ourselves better. I am not sure we always do, though.

Hemi Gilberg. 10 September 2018. Requiescat in pace.

* * *

'Hey, paths!' Richard Coutts boomed as he came into our laboratory. 'Got a curly one for you!'

'What's up, Richard?' I asked.

'I've just seen Stephanie Francis, who's as skinny as a rake with a pregnant-looking abdomen. She's already in her sixties, so that's out. The medicos saw her and decided to plunge a needle in to drain her belly of ten litres of fluid and, not surprisingly, that put her into shock. The ICU boys sorted that out, plus some pneumonia she got, and after a very rocky recovery, they sent her back to the ward. The physicians still decided she had a malignant ascites so they flicked her to the hospice for terminal care.'

'What did we diagnose on the fluid from the abdomen? Was it malignant?'

'No. You thought it was inflammatory.'

I nodded. We would have examined the fluid and done specialist immunohistochemistry to look for hidden cancer cells, as we did on every patient.

'So why do they think it's malignant? Do they know where it came from?'

'The hospice crew won't have a bar of it. They reckon it's a benign ovarian cyst that's completely filling her abdomen and pushing her diaphragm up into her chest. Steph's gut is so full she can hardly breathe. And she's wasted away to nothing. I think she was only ever skinny before but you should see her now.'

He looked gloomy.

'I reckon they've handed her over to us surgeons to polish her off. She's a terrible surgical risk.'

'What do you want us to do, Richard?'

'Can you check again and make sure it's not cancer? If it is, then we won't have to do a hopeless operation and knock her off. But if it's clearly benign … then who knows? I suppose I'll give it a go.'

'We'll check the slides again.'

We did, and it was still benign.

'How often does it look benign when it's actually malignant?' Richard asked thoughtfully.

'Almost never.'

Steph's husband, Glen, told me their story from the beginning. 'It didn't add up. They pushed a needle in and drained the fluid and she just collapsed. I waited for days outside of that ICU. Eventually the specialists told me to call in the family fast as she was on her way out. They came from all over. Some from Dunedin, and our son even rushed home from Amsterdam. We kept telling her: "Hold on, Chris comes back tonight. You just have to hold on for him." We all got there in the end. And then she didn't die. She even improved enough to be sent back to the ward. I thought the worst was over. Things would get better now. I had had lymphoma myself before and gone through chemotherapy and radiation, so I know how it works. Then it happened again. In the ward, they told me Steph was at the end of the line and they would have to refer her to the hospice for terminal care. She was going to die and there was nothing they could do. I just knew this wasn't right.'

Glen took Steph home to care for her. He moved her from their big house on Albert Street to a small, two-roomed unit at the back which was better to manage. They were destined never to return to their home. The family gathered protectively around — a salt-of-the-earth, lovely Kiwi family there for their mother and their grandmother's last scene in this world.

'Then this small bloke comes up the drive,' Glen said. 'Says he's head of the hospice and he's come to see Steph. Never had a doctor do a house call before.'

He shook his head in wonder. I wasn't surprised. The doctor was Simon Allan, the best palliative care doctor in the Manawatu and, we here are all sure, in the entire world.

'You're supposed to be dead, not lying there,' Simon said in his gentle Scots burr.

'I'm far too much of a bitch to die,' Stephanie retorted. The fiery response was fully in character for this woman.

Simon came and explained Steph's case to us as he saw it, which is what doctors do if things don't fit or the disease isn't doing what it should. They come and ask us to look again to see if there's anything we've missed.

'I don't think she has a malignant cancer. I think it's an ovarian cyst. She's desperately trying to exercise. She's eating incredibly well. And she seems to be gaining condition to me though she's still severely bloated. When did anyone with advanced cancer do that?'

Simon promised Steph and Glen that he would have a word to Richard Coutts to see what he could do. And here Richard was, asking the same questions. Had we missed anything?

We checked and checked again and we were sure. Everything we could see was absolutely benign. But benign or malignant, Steph's life hung in the balance.

After our conversation, Richard examined Steph for himself and reached a decision.

'I've had a brutal discussion with Glen and Steph Francis today,' he reported. 'She will die if we leave her as she is. Her ovary tumour is now causing such huge pressure effects on the belly that she's fading out. The medics made an ill-fated attempt to drain this in September, but not surprisingly, she went into shock. She's now worried that if we try anything else on her, it will produce the same result. That may be, but we have no choice.'

Richard told us how he had explained the outcome as he saw it to the Francis family. He's always an optimist.

'Your ovarian cyst is now in the terminal phase,' he told Steph. 'I reckon you've got a 50 per cent chance of dying on the table, but you'll have a long and fruitful life ahead of you if we can pull this off. I've had one other woman with this exact problem 20 years ago and we performed the procedure on her because her doctor objected strongly to her being sent to the hospice to die. I'll snatch out your cyst, too, but,' he glared at Stephanie pointedly, 'don't you go dying on me and spoiling my averages.'

Of course, whether he could operate or not depended entirely on whether he could find an anaesthetist to touch her case. Stephanie was so wasted away as to be skeletal. The hospital dietician said that she might have weighed 64.5 kilograms, but she looked closer to 30 to 40 kilograms, such was the degree of her muscle wasting. Her abdomen was so swollen that her crushed lungs laboured to draw breath. Steph posed a catastrophic risk under anaesthetic.

Richard turned to his long-suffering anaesthetist, Alberto Ramirez. This was a complex case, but Alberto was the natural choice, if only because Alberto's kids had been knocking around with Steph's for years. And Alberto is cut from the same adventurous cloth as Richard Coutts himself. He's Spanish and has the flair and exuberance of the Iberian folk. Perhaps he's suited by national temperament to have a go where others would run away. You also couldn't work alongside Richard for long without gaining an appetite for reaching out way past the surgically improbable towards the impossible.

Alberto rose to the challenge, although God only knew how this would all end.

'He told me I had to exercise and get fitter if I was to have any chance,' Steph told me. 'I had to eat and gain weight. My tumour might be benign, they said. Really? I would do it.'

Steph had that fundamental Kiwi toughness burning in her beautiful eyes.

'You have to have that determination just to carry on. It's inside of you,' Stephanie explained to me. 'I've always told my children that they have to be strong. Now I had to walk the talk. I exercised every hour of every day that I could. I skipped and exercised until I thought I would die of that instead. I ate everything that the dieticians wanted me to. And then I went up to the hospital. I was now in better shape than I'd ever been. I saw Alberto and I actually ran up to him, dancing up and down. He looked at me without knowing who I was and then his face lit up into a smile as he recognised me. "Stephanie! It's you! It's wonderful! You're ready now!"'

'This is going to be tricky,' Richard said. 'It's already touch and go at best. I'll do the bare minimum to get the cyst out and close up fast. I really should take out her uterus and the other fallopian tube and ovary, but I'll have to leave them alone this time.'

He looked regretful. Richard loves surgery. I think he regards any faintly suspicious organ as a surgical objective and to leave one behind is to walk away from a challenge.

Alberto planned the anaesthetic procedure with great care. It was the key to success.

'You'll have to operate with Steph on her left side and the first thing we'll do is very slowly drain the fluid so I can get some space for her lungs to ventilate into,' he told Richard.

'Can't we turn her onto her back after we've decompressed the cyst? I'd really prefer to operate with her like that.'

'No, too risky. You'll have to get it out operating from her side.'

'Okay. I'll have to bend over and it'll be strange but I won't be in there long. That much, I promise you! But you can bet that if she survives me on the table there'll be big fluid shifts and she'll go into respiratory failure like the last time they drained it.'

Alberto nodded. 'Stephanie has to go directly to ICU and be carefully managed. The odds of her going bad are high. The ICU want a termination-of-life plan before they'll take her on, of course.'

'Pessimists!' Richard snorted.

I wondered how Alberto was feeling about all this. I've personally always regarded anaesthetics as a terrifying responsibility for a doctor. For me, to render a person unconscious, then paralyse them and then assume responsibility for their very breathing is a shocking prospect. It makes me so grateful I can escape back to my own quiet world of pathology whenever I ponder it.

The day of the operation dawned. Alberto had to carry out extensive preparations to make sure that everything was as easy as it could be to keep Steph alive for the few minutes that Richard's surgery would take and the perfect storm that must follow her body losing 25 kilograms of fluid. All this planning took time and Richard hovered around anxiously, watching over Alberto's shoulder, offering unwanted suggestions.

'Go away, Richard!' Alberto snapped. 'I'll call you when I'm ready!'

Richard took it all in good humour. 'I took myself off,' he told me. 'The whole thing was all quite an elaborate anaesthetic exercise, really. I was only invited in for a short period and permitted to carry out some minimal surgery.'

* * *

An exuberant Richard raced into our lab. He was dressed as usual in his blue theatre scrubs. The grooves from the ties of his surgical mask decorated the sides of his face. His eyes sparkled. He was carrying a large plastic basin which he heaved with an obvious effort onto my desk. It was filled to the brim with bottles and bottles of murky, opalescent fluid. 'She's made it off the table, all credit to Alberto and his rejuvenation programme,' Richard crowed. 'That's the fluid we pulled off before starting. I've brought it here for you to have a play with. See if there's any malignancy. But those are for fun. I've got the real beast here.'

The cyst slouched in the bottom of the basin, trapped in a plastic bag like a caged animal. We looked with interest. It was a cream-coloured beach ball whose surface was coursed with a complicated meshwork of fine red vessels. It glared malevolently back at us like a bloodshot eye.

'Pretty, isn't it?' Richard was in his usual post-surgical euphoria. 'I met Glen in the corridor bringing this stuff from theatre. I think he was surprised to see me there with her bits. I let him have a dekko. I think he was impressed.'

The cyst weighed in at just over 12 kilograms, but most of it had already been drained away so we worked out that the intact cyst was something like 25 kilograms of alien occupying Steph's stomach. Steph only weighed in at 64.5 kilograms so nearly 40 per cent of her weight was cyst! The shrewd dieticians at the hospital had guessed correctly that she was mainly made of tumour.

Against the odds, Stephanie rallied strongly and recovered well. Of course, she had a lot of redundant skin left with that vast cyst out.

'I believe you should be a pin-up girl for the Shar-Pei dog society, as your abdominal skin suitably represents that breed,' Richard cheerfully told her. He gently prodded what remained, and looked at her hopefully. 'Of course, I could carve it off for you. Just a small nip and tuck?'

'No, thanks. I've had enough surgery to last me a lifetime. I'll just be a happy Shar-Pei puppy.'

'Well, you must contact the hospice and get an honourable discharge from their service. Now that's something that doesn't happen very often, does it? They can now add curing people to their showreel. We can only be thankful for their reluctance to reach straight for the euthanasia needle.'

It's interesting that Steph's affliction was a benign cyst. Benign things can kill you swiftly if they are in the wrong place, just as some highly malignant tumours never do anything or even just go away. Life, like Lotto, is full of chance and of the unexpected.

Stephanie and Glen live in a wonderful house decorated by beautiful murals visible from the end of the street. Your heart lightens as you approach, and you're glad to be welcomed by this family who went through so much and, especially, to see the irrepressible, lovely Stephanie, who clawed her way back from the very brink of death. For all its disappointments and frustrations, medicine can deliver some great results and moments of pure joy. Stephanie Francis is one.

Stephanie Francis
Mr Richard Coutts
Dr Alberto Ramirez
Dr Simon Allan
Valete! We salute you all!

* * *

'Have you heard, Doc? There's been another bombing in the States.'

'No! What happened?'

The events of 9/11 were still vivid in our minds, despite the 12 years that had rolled past.

'At the Boston Marathon. Two bombs have killed and injured a whole lot of people.'

Here we go again, I thought wearily. The world is full of madness and nothing is straightforward any more.

Pat was shaking his head as he checked the sharpness of my knife with his thumb and carefully laid it beside the instruments and sponge on the dissection table. It was a needless gesture, as he had personally honed it on the grinder.

A whole body 'pluck' lay beside the tools on the wooden board waiting for me. The patient's tongue and gullet hung over the edge framed by her carotid arteries. The lungs and the heart were face-down and the aorta lay sturdily between the two fat pads encasing the kidneys. The liver, spleen and stomach were completely hidden away beneath.

Blood dripped slowly from the severed arteries of the pelvis and darkly pooled around the tissues.

On one of the gurneys, her body shell lay empty, awaiting the return of its organs to their rightful place. But unlike the world, my patient was straightforward: a heart attack in a woman who had a history of atheroma affecting all three of her coronary arteries.

Boring. I looked at the second gurney, where Alex and her assistant Jackie were examining the body of a young man. He was short and stocky, obviously carrying some extra weight. There was something puzzling about his appearance, but I couldn't put my finger on it. He looked as if he would be medically far more interesting than my case.

'Isn't his abdomen a bit blown up?' I asked Alex. 'Has he got intestinal obstruction?'

'Could be. I thought that was because of central obesity. He's only 59 kilograms, though. He's a little overweight but not really obese.' Alex crouched and studied the profile of his dome-shaped gut from the side.

'No, I still think it's only central fat,' she decided, shaking her head.

'What's his story?'

We always need the whole story right at the beginning, if we're to make sense of our autopsy findings. Sometimes we're given all the facts, beautifully collected and in a logical order, and it makes our job so much easier. Other times, there's just not much there, and sometimes the critical part needed for the final diagnosis is missing altogether.

'Peter has Prader-Willi Syndrome.'

That would explain his build. I looked again at his body. Yes, I could see it now that my eye was attuned to the correct cues.

'Can you remind me of what that involves?'

'It's genetic, a chromosome-15 abnormality, and there is mild to moderate intellectual impairment. Peter has been living in supported accommodation with carers watching out for him. Prader-Willi sufferers typically have voracious appetites and their hunger is never, ever satisfied. So they eat and eat and will become morbidly obese unless they're controlled. And they can get diabetes, too, from their obesity. Peter's food is normally locked up to keep it away from him. Even the fridges have locks on them. Peter stole the keys from the carer and two nights ago broke into the pantry and the freezer. We don't know exactly what or how much he ate that night, but it was a lot.'

Alex picked up her notes and studied them.

'So far, they believe at least three complete loaves of bread, eight buns and 24 muesli bars have gone. There's a lot of food missing from the freezer, but they don't know what was there before and so how much he actually ate.'

'It seems unbelievable. How can you possibly fit all that in?'

'He did, but he didn't. Fit it all in, I mean. He vomited massively all over his bed and went dozens of times to the toilet. But the carer didn't twig and it was only the next morning that he saw Peter was in trouble. Apparently he was having difficulty walking. He could only waddle a bit. And of course, his stomach was huge and he was having trouble breathing. He was still vomiting everywhere, including some blood by then. So they took him to his GP. He ordered an X-ray of his abdomen, but he became so bad while they were doing it that he was then rushed to hospital by ambulance. He collapsed there suddenly and died while on the table having his CAT scan done.'

'Have we got the scan? That'd be the best evidence of the underlying pathology.'

'No, but we can get hold of it. And there's a report on it somewhere here in his hospital notes.'

Alex searched through the bulging folder. Peter was obviously well known to the hospital with many, many admission papers from down the years.

'Here it is.' Alex read it out to us. 'The chest shows poor air entry because of compression from significant abdominal distension. There is massive distension of the stomach, which is distended by food. There is also moderate gaseous distension of the small bowel and parts of the colon.'

'It seems pretty decisive,' I said, buffeted by a mild sense of déjà vu. It was like Hemi all over again. 'Gastric dilatation. Is he on any anti-psychotic drugs? Clozapine, perhaps?'

'Yes, but not clozapine. He's on risperidone.'

'What for? Is he bipolar, too?'

'It reduces his irritability and also helps damp down obsessive-compulsive disorders. Did you know Prader-Willi people are endlessly picking at their skin? And then there's their eating obsession, too. It helps stop both.'

'Hmm, I wonder if risperidone could cause gastric dilatation. Like the clozapine did with Hemi?'

'Prader-Willi patients are known to have episodes of gastric distension, but it's not understood if it's the disorder doing it or just the quantity of food they eat. Or maybe it's both? There are reports of it killing them, too.'

'Let's open him up and have a look, shall we?'

Peter's stomach was distended with gas but it wasn't really much more than we often see at autopsy anyway in patients who have had vigorous cardiopulmonary resuscitation. During mouth-to-mouth resuscitation, air is often forced down the oesophagus. Air-filled stomachs, together with many fractures of the ribs and the sternum, are signs a pathologist must know and recognise. They're an irrelevant product of well-meant activity that occurs only after life is extinct. Peter had both ribs and breastbone broken by the determined cardiac massage given in the hospital. They couldn't resurrect him, but it was effective, for we later found fragments of bone marrow embedded in vessels in his lungs, driven into the bloodstream from the rib fractures. This, too, is common and simply means that the massage was effective enough to keep the blood flowing. Old pathologists have learned to ignore bone marrow emboli.

But Peter's stomach was surprisingly small, although there certainly was still quite a lot of unrecognisable, soupy food in there, too. We gathered around and stared at the abdominal contents lying in the opened body before us. There didn't seem to be enough to compress the lungs. The distension had been there on the X-ray, for certain. Where had it gone?

Alex phoned the Emergency Department, found the specialist anaesthetist who had carried out Peter's resuscitation and explained the puzzle.

'I know what happened,' he explained. 'During the CPR, he vomited huge amounts of dark liquid vomit. And a lot of gas was pushed out, too. I reckon it was litres and litres. Maybe even as much as ten. That's where it's gone. Sorry, I should have put that down in his history.'

Without the complete history and the X-ray evidence, we would have been stumped. The diagnosis and the cause of death would have been a lot more difficult, if not impossible.

'There must have been a lot in there to start with. He was vomiting all night, too, so he would have vomited out quite a lot of what he ate through the night. And then add in ten litres expressed out at the resuscitation …'

It now added up.

Alex agreed. 'The distension must have been pretty enormous to make him as short of breath as he was reported to be. Still, it seems to me his distress and breathlessness seem almost out of proportion. I wonder if he has also aspirated food?'

Alex is a clever pathologist, always looking, evaluating and thinking. 'Does it fit? Does it make sense? Is there another explanation?'

A few days later, Alex passed me a microscope slide.

'Look at the histology of his lungs!'

She was right. There were bits of vomited food stuck in the airways and they had been there for many hours, as there was already a pneumonia around most of the chunks and the stomach acid had devitalised the bronchioles into a necrotic mush. Peter, in the stress of the all-night vomiting bout that followed his phenomenal binge, had inhaled both food and gastric acid straight into his lungs. That is an unhappy mix and would explain his severe distress and his rapid deterioration.

'It would take several hours before he died to get this degree of change,' I said quietly. 'He must have died pretty hard, I think.'

'Prader-Willi patients have a very high threshold for vomiting and for pain.' Alex had researched this subject carefully. 'That's a problem, because they'll eat spoiled and contaminated food but they're able to put up with a lot and only show up late in the disease.'

I've always had a soft spot for people with Prader-Willi, because I'm friends with a man who has this disorder. For a quarter of a century, I have met Chris by the river where we both walk our dogs. He's devoted to his dog and always knows the names of all the other dogs along the track. His dogs always have lovely personalities and I'm sure that's because he cares for them so well. I always understood that the aberrant genes conferred a mental impairment, but I can't see much of that in Chris. Medicine has always been really good at measuring disabilities but not really so quick to outline unconventional abilities. Chris had an amazing ability with numbers, patterns and figures. Probably it's all quite functionless, but it's impressive nonetheless.

'When were you born?' he challenged me one day.

'First of March, 1954.'

'Monday,' he snapped back, without even a fractional delay.

He was right, of course. This may not be hard to work out if you know how, but for the intellectually impaired? Oddly, too, people with Prader-Willi are known to be brilliant at jigsaw puzzles, though how and why certainly is a mystery.

Our genes are odd things but they are who we are. Peter was a victim of his genes and literally ate himself to death. He could no more help what happened to him than I can help having blue eyes. Of course, you don't need to have Prader-Willi syndrome to compulsively overeat. Many people overeat and some are compelled to do so. My Labrador dogs have all been compulsive eaters, and that is because many of them have a fat gene called POMC. This gene means they can't turn off their feeling of hunger, even when full. The gene also occurs in people where it does exactly the same thing and causes obesity.

And then, of course, there are the many of us who have a flair for eating pretty comprehensively, if not exactly compulsively, but without the excuse of any known genetic aberration. Many folk can and often do eat themselves to morbid obesity these days, and it's all their own work. Why is this?

I wondered about this when I performed an autopsy on a young girl. Julia was only 18 but she weighed 200 kilograms and was completely bedridden. Death is not uncommon in this situation, for a large number of complex metabolic reasons as well as infections and ulcers from the sheer weight of lying endlessly on your skin. The cause of death is not what puzzled me.

Her family were professional people and were highly skilled and intelligent. They carried trays of food in relays to Julia, even as she became too large to rise. Why did they do this? They were all of normal build themselves. Why couldn't they see what they were doing? There must be a compelling psychological reason behind this. The problem must be much bigger than just bad eating habits and a lack of exercise.

None of these factors were relevant to Peter's very sad and unfortunate death. The coroner heard all the evidence and was critical of the carers for under-reporting the amount Peter had eaten and for not acting faster when he first became unwell. I understood that, well enough, and it was true that things could have been done better. But I thought afterwards that caring for the intellectually impaired, however mild the impairment might be, must be a thankless task, and to protect those they care for from every potential harm, every hour of every day, is a hard ask of anyone.

Peter. Requiescat in pace.

EPILOGUE

—and the Dead

Who will give and account to Him that is ready to judge the Quick and the Dead?
—1 Peter 4:5

We have sanitised and medicalised death in our modern Western society.

When a loved one dies, the police may be notified if it is unexpected, a doctor will examine the body and pronounce that life is extinct, whereupon an undertaker will whisk the body away to a mortuary for an autopsy or to a funeral home to be fitted for a coffin. The family and friends are kept at a distance and the absence of the body is oddly seen as a sign of deep respect. We are now a largely secular society, with few religious beliefs or rituals to apply to the dead to assist their journey to the afterlife.

This is not quite true of Maori. We do our utmost to return the tupapaku — the bodies of the dead — to their whanau on the day of death so they can sit with their loved ones and mourn them properly. Most Kiwis have had some contact with the more natural Maori attitude to death, and this is a positive thing in our culture.

The great-hearted Hawke's Bay coroner Chris Davenport told me of an elderly Maori woman who came to see him. Her late husband was lying in the back of the ute parked outside.

'His heart has killed him. He's had trouble for years,' she explained. 'He just wouldn't listen. I told him, "Go and see the doctor! You need pills!" But he wouldn't listen. I put him in the ute and drove him here myself and he saw the doctors down at the medical centre. They said it was his heart and gave him pills for his heart. I knew it! But he threw them out the window when we were driving back. And now he's dead. The doctors said they weren't surprised and gave me a certificate. But I have a question.'

'What is it?' Chris asked in his quietly compassionate way.

'My aunties say it's illegal. Is it illegal to bury a body without a coffin?'

'No,' Chris said. 'You have a death certificate. That's all you need. You don't need a coffin.'

'Thank you so much!'

She seized and hugged Chris. He was that sort of man. She turned to leave.

'What will you do now?' Chris asked.

'I'm going to get a spade, take him back up into the bush and bury him under a tree,' she replied.

I thought about that for a bit. 'What did you say?' I asked Chris.

Chris smiled. 'I didn't say anything. I just couldn't bring myself to tell her that *that* was actually illegal. I just watched her drive off.'

* * *

In our Western society, the very words associated with 'death' are sanitised, too.

'If something should happen to me ...' people will say. What on earth do they mean? What is that 'something' to which they are referring? What they mean to say is 'If I die ...'

But even that is wrong, for it's not the 'if' for any living creature. It's 'when'.

'He passed away,' they might say. Or: 'He went to sleep and never woke up again.' No, he didn't do either of those things. He died. Why do we hide so from the language of death?

This mixed rhetoric reminds me of the Irish nuns who nursed me during my tonsillectomy at Saint Anne's Hospital. I was only eight years old and in those days you were hospitalised for a full week for that particular operation. Each night, when they came to pray over us and turn down the lights, they would admonish us, saying: 'Be sure to say your prayers tonight for fear that you should wake up dead in the morning!'

Death.

I have to confess that I am an aficionado of death. I am fascinated by all aspects of death and the dead and I suppose that's why I am so fortunate to have landed up in my particular profession. Wherever I have travelled in the world, I have sought out the dead and their stories and looked at how the locals treat them.

Elayne and I drove from Spoleto in Italy to the quaint commune of Ferentillo, with twin fortifications on the opposite sides of the hills in the Valnerina river valley. It's a bit off the beaten track, but it's home to what is now

—and the Dead

apparently the most visited museum in Umbria, the Museum of Mummies. It hadn't been discovered when we went, all those years ago. It was somnolent, possibly because it was high noon and the townspeople's *riposo* time. I had to bang on an ancient wooden door, where eventually a very large, mediaeval-looking key was grumpily handed over and we were directed to the crypt of the Church of Santo Stefano.

We let ourselves in, quite unsupervised, and looked around in disbelief. There were dozens of beautifully preserved, dried, mummified bodies, mostly hundreds of years old and still dressed in their original and ancient clothes. There was a Chinese honeymoon couple in their finest attire. The groom was in a formal suit, as befitted a gentleman of that time. These two had died of cholera while on their tour in 1750 and were laid to rest here. I find that amazing. Did they really come all the way from China in a sailing ship, two and three-quarter centuries earlier? Why did they do that? What did their folk think when they didn't come back? What happened to their wedding gifts? And their home? My mind just churns with these unanswered questions.

There, in the crypt, also lies the local bellringer of 200 years ago. He fell from his tower and still has the crudely closed cuts from an autopsy visible on his neck. Who was the pathologist, I wonder? Was it just the local surgeon. What did he discover? Was it a broken neck?

And oddly, there is a mummified eagle in there with its wings outstretched, glaring balefully at you. The bird died and was placed for some reason in the crypt, where he, too, has mummified.

Why did the extraordinary preservation of all these bodies even happen?

That one, at least, I can answer. The conditions of the crypt are perfect for mummification. There is a warm, dry wind that blows steadily up the valley and enters the crypt through three lancet windows, creating the ideal temperature and humidity. The wind also bears a fine mist of fungal spores and these produce an antibiotic that kills off the bacteria of decay. And some think the rich blend of minerals in the soil may help, too. Or maybe it is just the will of God, as the locals have believed for centuries.

There is also an *ossario* there, where the bones of dozens of skeletons remain interred on hallowed ground. The presence of these bones is also explicable. The early Eastern Church Christians would bury their dead for up to three years and then publicly disinter them to establish their purity. In his well-researched novel *Birds Without Wings*, Louis de Bernières tells the story of Polyxeni, who is present at her mother Mariora's exhumation three years after her death. She's frightened, for the exhumation doubles as an inquiry into moral character during life, and Mariora had a certain reputation. The idea was that if the person were sinful, then the earth would reject their flesh. If, however, all her flesh was gone and only her skeleton remained, her innocence would be demonstrated. Based on the results of this important trial, it was then decided where your body was to be buried.

The women of the village all watch carefully as Mariora's skull is lifted from the soil and the earth prised from the eye sockets. The clean skull is lifted, teeth gently pushed back into their sockets and the forehead is reverently kissed. The earth has received her well, for there is no flesh and Mariora is free of sin. Her bones will now be placed in the church ossuary. Mariora will now spend eternity lying in hallowed ground within a church, and will not be burned or reburied in an unconsecrated and lonely grave, the fate of the sinful.

There are hundreds of these ossuaries scattered throughout Europe. In the Orthodox monasteries, the bones of monks were dug up and stored in aptly named charnel houses. The biggest ossuary I have seen is in the Catacombs of Paris. Here, spread over three acres, are the beautifully arranged bones of six million Parisians. The graveyards were filled to overflowing in the 1700s and so it was decreed that the graves should be opened, the skeletons exhumed and stored in the catacombs. The tunnels cover about 300 kilometres and the bones are arranged in sets of skulls, of femurs and of ribs and every bone in between.

I was intrigued to find on closer examination that some had obvious holes from musket balls, others had badly healed fractures and I found a couple with tumours. I would need my microscope and a slide to say whether the tumours were malignant sarcomas or were infectious tuberculomas or even syphilitic gummas. The men who laid the bones there were artists and the skulls particularly are arranged in lovely patterns, including one wall where they are beautifully arranged to form a heart. Behind these artistic façades, there are millions more bones lying in disorderly piles, just as they were dumped hundreds of years ago.

It is a very odd thing to find beneath the streets of a lovely, vibrant modern city like Paris. A visit there is not for the faint-hearted, though, so be warned. My daughter Charlotte felt distinctly uneasy and was relieved to reach the other side and exit into the fresh air beneath the blue sky.

In Salta, Argentina, we went to see the Inca child mummies left to die of cold at the summit of Llullaillaco, 22,000 feet up in the Andes, as *qhapaq hucha*, or living sacrifices. There were three bodies available for us to see and they remain almost perfectly preserved, looking much as they did when they were first put up there in 1550. There are two sisters: La Doncella, a 15-year-old virgin sacrifice, and the six-year-old La Niña del rayo. The younger girl shows the scorch marks typical of a lightning strike to her face and ears. This would have happened some time during the hundreds of years they lay there undisturbed. The girls were peacefully at rest, but the seven-year-old boy, El Niño, seemed to me to have died hard. He alone of the three is tied up. I think he was frightened and must have tried to run down after the priests when they left him behind to die. They then had no choice but to tie him up and leave him there. He has vomited down his front, but whether that was from fear or during the process of dying from the cold, I cannot say.

I found the study of their DNA and that of the many other sacrificial children who have been discovered equally fascinating. One lad's mitochondrial DNA profile, which he inherited from his mother, is so rare that it has been found in only three modern-day people in all of South America. Yet it once was a common gene in the people who lived there. The guns and diseases of the Spanish conquistadors spared no-one. Of 84 separate genetic lineages identified from a collection of these mummies and skeletons, not one single modern-day living person has been found anywhere in South America. This speaks volumes of how completely an entire nation and culture was wiped out in the atrocity of colonisation. These dead are still here today, the silent witnesses to us, the living, of the tragedy that befell their people all those long, long centuries ago.

—and the Dead

In Japan, I learned of the personal respect they accord their dead. The *yukatas* — ceremonial garments — worn by the dead are closed right over left, while the living wear theirs left over right. This fun fact is one useful thing for Western tourists who dress up to go to the public baths to know. You don't want to go to the baths and be thought of as a zombie, do you? The body is then lightly cremated and the relatives will gather around the ashes and reverently pick up the bones with metal chopsticks. The chopsticks are held vertically, and that's why it is considered impolite to hold chopsticks like that when eating food. Two relatives often pick up and hold one piece of bone together in an act they call *kotsuage*. That's the only time it's permissible to do this, and why you never, ever pass food from chopsticks to chopsticks at a meal. The bones of the dead are gently placed in an urn in an orderly way with the foot bones first and those of the skull last.

There are other exotic rituals of death that I have heard of but never seen. Parsis in India, who follow the Zoroastrian religion, have always put their dead on top of Towers of Silence, where vultures would dispose of the bodies in minutes. This practice has declined since the 1990s, as 99 per cent of the vultures have been wiped out by poisoning from the diclofenac used to treat livestock.

A similar 'sky burial' is also practised by Tibetan Buddhists, who place their dead upon mountaintops for the holy condors and other carrion birds to eat. It is an effective method of excarnation or de-fleshing a body, and is seen as a sign of generosity to other forms of life. It was a practice that Mao Zedong abhorred and was determined to stop as part of his critical modernisations. It still occurs, but much less frequently. I would very much like to see a sky burial, but I know I never shall — not because they are so very rare, but out of respect for the dead. Strangers are not allowed at the ceremony, as it is believed that their presence will significantly diminish the transmigrating soul.

Respect for the dead underpins all these customs, and that's what I have seen everywhere I have been. It is amazing that humans handle their dead in so many different ways. Whether they are in an open casket at a tangihanga with the tupapaku there to sit by, or the bones are picked out of the ashes with chopsticks or the body taken to the heavens on the wings of a holy condor, it is the same. Everything we do for our dead is done out of honour and respect for them. I try to keep that front and centre in my mind, every day that I put on my gown and mask and my surgical gloves and seek to ask a body for the answers to the questions that their death has posed.

Death twitches my ear. 'Live!' he commands
   'For I am coming.'
   — Virgil (70–19 BC)